Fat and Fed Up, No More!

Catherine Hassett

Fat and Fed Up, No More!
7 Steps to Permanent Natural Weight Loss

Copyright © 2011 by I CAN Coaching Publishing.

Edited by Kay Watt

Second Edition 2012

British Library Cataloguing Publication Data.
A catalogue record for this book is available from the British Library

ISBN: 978-0-9569738-1-8

Published by
I CAN Coaching Publishing
Ireland

Nota Bene:

I have made every effort in this book to present the information as accurately as possible. The majority of the information is based on my learning from my Life Coaching Diploma and my personal and professional experience.

This content of this book is set out in good faith, for general guidance on your journey to achieving permanent natural weight loss. It is intended to complement, not to replace, any professional medical, nutritional or fitness advice that you may need on this journey.

What you put into this book and the tasks is what you will get out of it. Naturally, I cannot guarantee your results, nor be held responsible for any actions that you may take as a consequence of implementing the tools and strategies set out in this book.

Also please note; No part of this book may be reproduced or transmitted in any form whatsoever, without written permission from the author, except for the inclusion of brief quotations in a review.

Contents

For my loving husband Derek,
whose belief in me,
helps me to believe "I CAN".

Thank You!

To Halina,
for all your help and positivity.
Ich bin Ihnen sehr dankbar.

Foreword by Martin Fitzgerald

We have known for over a decade that over half of our body's immune system is in our gut and that the intestines have more nerve connections than the spinal cord. It comes as a surprise to most people to know that there are more bacterial cells in our gut than human cells in our whole body.

The old joke among biologists is to ask the question;

> "Who is the host? Are the bacteria living on us or are we living on the bacteria?".

They are responsible for breaking down the building blocks that make our bodies work and heal. They influence the rate of food break-down and absorption. As a result they affect our energy levels and consequently our tolerance, patience and will power, to name just a few emotional responses.

If we are what we eat then certainly the concept of "we think what we eat" can't be too far behind. What we eat affects what we think; conversely what we think affects what we eat. We always focus on our food diet, but how many of us have looked at our psychological diet? What do we feed our brains?

We live in a time of idealised expectation. From the time we watch Cinderella in Disney cartoons as children, to fashion shows as teenagers and into our 20's; the media bombardment throughout our whole life is for this or that 'In thing'. As happiness is a function of expectation they set us up for an inevitable fall. One fall after another! This creates the perfect consumer – always feeling being behind, not good enough – needing something to fill the gap between where we are and where they tell us where we should be. The solution is always only a few bucks away. That outfit, that exercise machine, that diet. Until we eventually realise that it doesn't work and we have to spend more yet again. And again!

Some continue along this yellow brick road of illusion. Others stop and think it out for a while. Even the most intelligent of people are caught up in it all because they are led to believe there are no other options. Actually, the other option is obvious. So obvious that it is staring you in the face every single day. We don't see it because it is so obvious. Why is our attention not brought to it? because there is no commercial gain in telling you. You don't have to spend money on this and it's one and final thing you have to do. There are no magic potions, fad diets or exercise routines.

Catherine Hassett leads you to the one place you may never have looked where the one and final successful solution is waiting; inside yourself.

Permanent weight loss is only one of the benefits from reading this book. The author lifts the veil of illusion and challenges you to take a look that you've been avoiding. You'll find that, actually what lies inside is the reality that you can deal with successfully; for weight and for life.

The author shows us that the rest of it all is just one big fairytale!

Martin Fitzgerald
MSc., Lic.Ac. (TCM), M.A.C.I.

Martin Fitzgerald is an experienced scientist from Ireland. Having spent over 12 years research and development work in colleges, universities and the pharmaceutical industry both in Ireland and the UK. He has published research in the area of food science and chemistry. Most recently assisting the EMEA (European Medicines Agency) and FDA (Food and Drug Administration of America) who included his work in the United States Pharmacopeia. He is also a qualified Chinese Medicine practitioner having studied in Ireland and China and runs private practices in Ireland.

Section 1:

The Introduction

Chapter 1:

Who is this book for?

This book is designed to help you to lose weight permanently, in a natural way, in 7 easy to follow steps.

You will find it extremely useful if:

- You are fed up with being overweight.
- Your body shape effects your self esteem.
- You feel unhappy, helpless, hopeless, self conscious, depressed, lonely, anxious, sad or angry because of your weight.
- You feel your weight is affecting your health.
- You feel out of control with your eating.
- You are sick and tired of trying to lose weight.
- You are fed up with yo-yo diets.
- You are tired of putting weight back on after a diet.
- You want to learn how to lose weight in a healthy way without dieting or using weight loss supplements or meal replacements.
- You want to free your mind of incessant thoughts about food, calories, points, weighing scales and eating.
- You want to be able to enjoy eating in a social situation.
- You want to have a healthy relationship with food and eating.
- You want to learn new ways of coping with difficulty and pain in your life that doesn't involve food.
- You want to eat without experiencing negative emotions like shame and guilt.
- You want to learn how to set goals and achieve them.
- You want to learn how to control your thoughts, feelings and behaviours.

- You want to learn how to make positive changes in your life.
- You want to experience more happiness, more contentment, more satisfaction, more joy, more fulfilment and more achievement in your life.

When I use the word fat, it is not as a label or a judgement. I believe fat is about how you feel, it doesn't matter if you are 7 lbs or 7 stone overweight. What it comes down to is how your body shape makes you feel. It is not about what society or anybody else says about it.

There are many people that may be a bit overweight, according to what society says they should weigh, but they live active healthy lives and they don't feel fat, they feel happy in themselves and the way they look. It is all based on how you feel inside.

This to me is the optimum place to be, a place where you are healthy and happy, both inside and out.

I cannot emphasise enough the importance of the role of your health in this process. I will never condone weight loss in an unhealthy way, or the loss of weight that causes ill-health. Being underweight affects your health and shortens your life just as much as being overweight. What is the point of achieving a body shape, that you think will make you happy, but instead you become so unhealthy you cannot enjoy your life? I have been down this road and I know my health is not at its optimum now because of my obsession with being thin when I was younger. If you are prepared to be thin at the cost of your health, please continue to read this book first and then make a decision about the best thing that you can do for you.

If you feel fat and it is affecting your life, your health and your happiness and you feel it is time for a change, a permanent natural change, then this book is for you.

Chapter 2:

How can this book help you?

This book is different to most of the weight loss books out there because it is designed to help you to actively help yourself. As you know, nobody can make you happy with your body shape and no one can lose the weight for you. It is all up to you; you are in complete control. However, because of what you may have experienced in the past, you may not feel like you are in complete control, or maybe even believe you ever could be. No matter what background you have, no matter what you have experienced in life, no matter what has caused you to gain weight or to be unhappy with your shape, this book will help you, to help yourself, to feel in complete control.

The power of this book lies in the use of Life Coaching techniques. Life Coaching is about empowering people so that they can achieve what they want and desire in life, by using their strengths, knowledge and skills. The Life Coach believes that every client has all the personal resources they need to solve their own problems.

People gain huge clarity and perspective in their lives through coaching and in turn this enables them to see clearly what they want out of life and how they can get it. They learn how to face the challenges and obstacles that life invariably throws their way and how to overcome them. They learn how to set clear and specific, achievable goals and decide on each step they need to take to achieve them.

This book is designed to be a self-coaching handbook, but one that I have written in combination with my personal and professional experience in weight loss and one that I have specifically formulated to help you to coach yourself to achieve happiness with your body shape.

You don't have the benefit of working face to face with a coach when using a book like this, but what you will get is a handbook that facilitates you to ask yourself the right questions, and enable you to find the right answers.

You will recognise your weaknesses as well as your strengths, enjoy your success and review what does not go to plan. You will also learn tools and techniques that will help you to be a very effective self-coach.

I must clarify however, that while I am a qualified Life Coach, I am not a nutritionist or a fitness expert and thus I do not give any advice on nutrition or exercise. If you need advice on either of these areas please ask a qualified professional.

No matter what your goal is, this book will help you to achieve it. It will help you to help yourself. Before you start I ask you to accept that you are here today because of the choices that you have made, without blame or guilt. Then make a promise and commitment to yourself that you are going to put in every ounce of energy that you have, to make these changes possible:

- ✓ If you are willing to give yourself the time and effort that you deserve to complete this book like it is intended;
- ✓ If you have the willingness to accept that you are responsible for your situation and your life as well as the desire to make the changes needed;
- ✓ Then you have everything you need to achieve your goals and realise your dreams.

Chapter 3:

The Author's Weight Loss Journey:

"They can because they think they can"

Virgil

I wrote this book because I have been Fat and Fed UP and I believe that I have something to say that may help others that feel that way too. I have had my weight on my mind for about 17 years of my life. I have tried diet after diet and yet failed to maintain or be happy with the result.

For half my life I have spent most of my waking hours thinking about food, weight, calories, thinness, burning off food intake, etc.

I know what it is like to be so unhappy with your body shape that it affects you in every area of your life. I know what it is like to be so obsessed with being thin that it consumes your thoughts. I know what it is like to constantly restrict yourself when eating. I know what it is like to feel hungry all the time, but to love the feeling because it means your body is being forced to use fat and burn calories. I know how losing weight the wrong way can damage your health.

I know how hard it is to lose weight. I know how difficult it can be to shake the bad habits. I know what it is like to go on a diet and lose some weight only to gain it all once the diet regime stops. I know what it is like to feel your life is just one big diet.

I know how being on a diet makes you think about all the things you are not allowed to have. I know how one indulgence or break out with "can't have" food on a diet can cause you to think "I have ruined it now, I may as well give up the diet".

I know how struggling with your weight can make you feel so many horrible emotions like frustration, shame, guilt, disappointment, despair and many more.

I know what it is like to have pain in your life.
I know what it is like to feel hopeless about your weight.

I could go on, but I will assume you can see what I am saying. Basically I have been there done it and got the T-shirt, varying in seizes from 16 to 10! In my late teens and early 20's I thought I had to be thin to be happy. So I achieved the skin and bone shape or near enough. This is difficult to maintain as it is not a natural state for your body. So over the following years I put on some weight, a lot to do with being young and enjoying my social life. On and off again I would think about my weight and restrict my eating to lose more weight.

Into my late 20's and early 30's I opted for actual diets. I would try one, find it awful or break out and give up. Then later, I would try another and the same thing would happen. The cycle would repeat itself diet after diet. I just got more fed up and frustrated.

The most I would ever carried over my ideal weight would be between 1 to 2 stone and for my height I was able to carry it. Many of my friends would say they never remember me being fat. This didn't matter to me, the fact was I felt fat and I was not happy.

My temporary freedom from thoughts about my weight and body shape came when I got pregnant. It was great. My body shape was going to change outside of my control, I could rest my mind from caring about it for a while and eat without thinking about the calories: I thought!

I gave up alcohol and tea and coffee and all the other things pregnant women are told to stay away from, but other than that I could eat freely. So I did.

Everything went fine; I gave birth to a beautiful baby boy at home, just as I had planned. It was a truly amazing experience. I couldn't have been happier.

That was until a few weeks after my son's birth when the scales told me I had gained three and a half stone. It was the heaviest I had ever been. My liberal eating had taken its toll. I was fat and very fed up! I hated myself in everything I wore, I avoided going out socially, I was absolutely miserable. The thoughts of more diets and restrictions made me feel worse.

It was at this time that it finally hit me. I had spent half my life obsessing about my weight and being unhappy with my body. I realised this wasn't healthy and definitely not a recipe for happiness. I decided I was not going to spend the rest of my life doing the same thing. It was time for a change, a real change. Not for another diet and horrible fitness regime that was torture to keep up, but a REAL change.

At this stage I was a qualified Life Coach and the answer was staring me in the face. It was time to practice what I preached. I knew nothing was going to work until I changed my beliefs, my relationship with and my attitude to food. I had to look at what I was eating and why I was eating it. I ditched the diets and worked on myself.

I set my goal. I had three stone to lose.
- I made changes to my lifestyle that I liked and that I chose, not what someone else told me to do.
- I did things because I wanted to, not because I thought I should.

- I knew what a healthy diet entailed and I knew it was important to move more when losing weight and also to be fit and healthy.

I started eating well and walking every day. I always loved walking and doing something you enjoy is a huge help. I timed my walks everyday with my son's sleep time. Pushing the pram while he slept gave us both what we wanted, and it worked perfectly into my routine.

But I also started to do something I had never done before, I started to eat consciously and I connected with my body. I would enjoy and savour every mouthful of food but when my stomach felt like it had enough I would stop eating. If my stomach was satisfied, my body had enough food at that time: I learned to trust this. Anymore food would be surplus to my body's requirements and it would be converted to fat, defeating what I was trying to achieve.

Over the years, I had lost the ability to trust my body. In the early years, I ignored it when it told me it was hungry and I forced it to feed on my reserves. Later I listened to someone else's ideas of when I should and should not eat, in the form of a diet.

I also discovered that I had irrational beliefs about body shape. I had bought into what our diet and body obsessed culture had been telling me. That changed too. It was time to bin those beliefs. Now I have new life enhancing beliefs that supported my goals in life. I decided that my happiness did not lie in the body shape that our culture decides is attractive and "right".

I believe now that my happiness lies in feeling healthy and fit, because it means that I can enjoy an active life with my family which is very important to me. We cycle, walk, climb mountains and swim because we love to do it. This is what makes me happy. I have come to accept my body. I am a healthy weight, I achieved my goal and exceeded it, I lost three and a half stone and I think I look good. I am not a size eight and I never will be and I never want to be. The life of restriction and diets and being unhappy with my body shape are behind me.

I don't deny myself anything and I don't feel guilt or anxiety around food, I enjoy what I eat. I can do this because I changed my thoughts. I connect with my body, I eat consciously and I use food for fuel. I can go out and enjoy a nice meal. If I feel like a dessert I will have one, if I don't I won't. Every decision I make about food now is a conscious one. I will check with my body and honour it, just as it deserves.

I maintain an active lifestyle doing the things that I enjoy and that make me feel good. I changed my irrational beliefs.

Now I know happiness comes from within, not from my body shape.

My happiness comes from living an active healthy lifestyle with my family, enjoying the company of my friends, seeing the positive and funny side of life, enjoying my work and from being grateful every day for all that I have in my life. This was a very important lesson I learned and one which I want to pass onto you.

Your weight is causing you to be unhappy now, possibly in most areas of your life and because of this you want to make a change by setting a goal and achieving it. However, there are many wonderful things in life today that can be enjoyed and bring you happiness. Try not to "put off" being happy until you achieve your goal. Don't lose today in pursuit of tomorrow.

This introduction tells you that I know how painful it can be to be fat; but I also know how wonderful and exhilarating it feels to achieve your desired body shape and to feel happy in it. I know what it is like to become that shape that you have wanted for a very long time. I know what it is like to take control of your life and achieve the freedom that comes with release from the prison of a fat body: I know the joy that comes with being happy in your own skin, in the shape of your choosing.

If you are thinking there is a lot about me in a book that is supposed to be helping you, you are right.

However, I am telling you all of this because I want you to know, that I know, what it is like to be fat and fed up, so much so that I decided to be Fat and Fed Up, No More!. My clients appreciate knowing I have some idea of what they are going through and they can also see that I have come through the other side. It is because of this, that I know this book will help you, if you give it the chance. Every technique I have described is one that I have used myself and that has worked and that work for my clients on a daily basis.

My heart is in this book, as well as my personal and professional experience. I am truly passionate about what I do. My passion lies in helping people to get to where they want to be with their body shape, once and for all, and helping them to experience the joy and exhilaration that come with achieving their goals.

Through my personal and professional experience I have developed tools, techniques and strategies that work and that I want to share with you. If this book can help one person to achieve happiness with their body shape and help them to create a healthy body and a healthy mind, then it was well worth writing.

- If you have tried diet after diet with no success;
- If you have reached a point where you feel like you have tried everything and nothing works;
- If you start believing "I will never lose weight"........

.... You are right! You will never lose weight, if you continue to do it the way you have been doing it up to now. You have proven to yourself that these ways do not work. It is time for a change, a new approach, and new techniques.

It is time to *be Fat and Fed Up, No More!*

The fact that you are reading this book implies that you might believe that maybe there is something that can help you. I believe there is something that can help you and I have written it down in the pages of this book.

The first thing that I want you to do is,

- Heed the words of the famous Roman poet, Virgil: *"They can because they think they can"*.

If you have some scepticism about this then it is completely understandable. Maybe you are thinking, "How can I believe that I can do this when every attempt I have made so far has failed? It goes against everything I have experienced to date."

Yes, this is a fair point, but I don't expect you to believe it to be true at this stage I just want you to *think* it.

There is a difference: believing something is having conviction about it; when you are convinced it is true, it becomes your belief. Thinking it on the other hand requires you to bring it into your conscious mind, merely as an idea.

What this will do, very powerfully, is help to change your focus, from what can't be done to what can be done. We will look at focus later in more detail, but for the moment if you put the thought "I CAN do this" into your head, you will start looking at ways to help you do it rather than ways to stop you.

You will start focusing on the possibilities rather than the obstacles. That's all it takes right now, it's just a thought. A small thought, but a thought that can help you to achieve so much. What have you got to lose? How much have you got to gain?

- The second thing you need to do is keep reading......

 I C A N C o a c h i n g P u b l i s h i n g

Chapter 4:

Are you ready to make a change?

**"Rather than wishing for change,
you first must be prepared to change"**

Catherine Pulsifer

"Fed Up" is defined as, "disgusted with" and "sick and tired of".

Are you fed up with how you look?

Are you fed up of trying diet after diet without achieving any long term results?

Are you fed up with counting calories?

Are you fed up with the eat-guilt-eat cycle?

Are you fed up carrying extra weight that seems impossible to shift?

Are you ready to say *Fat and Fed up, No More!?*

If you are ready to make changes once and for all that will bring you the results you want, then use this book to help you step by step, to release the real you from under that unwanted fat.

My situation may be similar or different to your experience, but whatever your situation is, the only way to lose weight and to keep it off is by addressing what is going on in your mind. You have to look at your habits and patterns, why you eat, your way of thinking about food, what you get from food outside of nourishment and much more.

Do this along with eating right and moving right and you will lose weight and keep it off. If you give your mind the workout that it needs, you can have it all, you CAN be thin and eat what you want and never have to think about dieting ever again.

Making changes however, can be difficult. When you have been doing things the same way for years, it takes work and courage to make the change to do those things differently. If you have been eating chocolate for years because you believe it helps you to cope with the stress in your life then it can be a very daunting task facing the possibility of a life without this form of stress release and comfort.

The key point to remember when facing a change like this, or any change for that matter, is without change nothing is going to improve. If the way you have been living up to now has not brought you to a good place where you are happy with your body shape, then you have been doing things the wrong way. Now it is time for you to find the right way.

While the thought of leaving your comfort zone might be a scary prospect, if you stay where you are now you are going to remain fed up. A positive change can bring you more happiness and joy.

Is it worth the effort? Is it worth *your* effort?

Chapter 5:

How to Use this Book:

In this book I will guide you through 7 steps, to permanent natural weight loss. I use life coaching techniques and strategies that will help you to make your own changes. These techniques and strategies are those that I use with my face to face clients every day. This book will help you to be your own coach.

The unique aspect of this book is that it will help you to create your very own self coaching manual. By completing the tasks I have set out for you, you will not only get in touch with your true self, your thoughts, and your emotions but you will also be creating a handbook of tools and strategies that are completely unique to you and your weight loss journey. It will act as a means of self analysis which will also work as a powerful tool. At the end of this book you will have your very own record of progress, which will contain many tools that you can dip into for help at any stage to take you to where you want to be.

In every chapter we will address a different topic in relation to weight loss the "I CAN" way. At the end of the chapter I will ask you to complete a task that makes the chapter specific to you. By completing these tasks you will learn more about yourself in relation to weight loss, but in ways that will help you in all areas of your life. Following these tasks I offer a strategy based on what you have learned. These strategies are designed to enable you to create a new, sustainable, healthy lifestyle that will ultimately bring you the happiness you seek.

Remember, you are working on habits and thoughts that you have possibly

---

spent years putting into place. These are not going to disappear overnight, but with practice and time your new thoughts and habits will become your new reality and your new way of living.

If, like me, you are the type of person who likes to flick to the end of a book just to see what kind of ending it is, or if you like to flick through a book and pick pieces from it here and there, I would urge you to avoid the temptation. The ending in this case is going to be entirely up to you. You are in complete control, you will be setting your own goal and you will decide whether you achieve it or not. Also reading the sections out of sequence will not serve any purpose.

This is developed to be a step by step approach, each step is essential in its own right. More importantly as a part of a process, each step is going to be more powerful because of the one you took before it.

Chapter 6:

My philosophy: the basis of this book

I believe there are 3 steps we need to take to lose weight and keep it off, they are:
1) *Think right,*
2) *Eat right*; and
3) *Move right.*

The combination of these 3 steps will enable you to achieve your goal and realise your dreams. Diets are not part of this process! They do not work, they serve only to create a psychology of denial and change your focus to what you CAN'T have.

Many of us that want to lose weight want a magic pill and want results yesterday! So we reach for the diets that promise to make us lose 10 lbs in 2 weeks, or the diet supplements that say they will shave 6 inches off our waists in no time, or the meal replacement shakes that promote fat loss in a simple shake. For most people these options do not work, because they are not realistic. Despite this however, we still go back for more. When one diet does not work we look for another. People still choose the same path that leads them back to the same place.

This is similar to the fly that repeatedly crashes into the window pane in his attempt to fly to freedom. He tries it numerous times but does not succeed. He persists in repeating the process over and over only to repeat his failure over and over. The fly with the mental capacity he was born with, is unable to learn from his many attempts and change his technique to achieve success. However, we as humans can!

- We can change our beliefs, our emotions and our behaviours because we have 100% control over them, even though we often think we don't, and;
- We can learn from our successes and mistakes.

These are a must when you want to lose weight for life!

I live my life by following 3 core principles:
   1) Learn from the past
   2) Look forward to the future
   3) Live in today

First of all, while coaching is mainly concerned with the present and the future, I believe there is a lot to be gained from looking to your past, especially when it comes to understanding weight issues and in assisting you to find the solutions. You might consider your past to contain many failures but they are not a waste if you learn something from them. In the future you will know how not to do something if it didn't work in the past.

Many people have the belief that because they failed to lose weight so many times in the past, that they are doomed to fail in the future. This is one of those generalisations that we tend to make. We are not failures because we failed to reach a goal. A goal, that was quite possibly unrealistic and one that was attempted using unrealistic means.

Secondly, by looking forward to the future you have new things to focus on and aspire to. My mother always called me a dreamer, but without dreams how do we know what we want? A question used regularly in coaching by the coach is,

"If there were absolutely no limitations in your life, no obstacles to stop you, what would you want to do?"

They are talking about a dream, something that would be amazing to achieve. So why not aspire to achieving it? There is only one thing that will stop you doing anything in your life and that is YOU!

Change the way you think about things, what you focus on and work on all those limiting beliefs that you have accumulated over the course of your life. Do that and you can realise your dreams.

Thirdly, live in today so you don't miss out on all the beauty and wonder and love that surround you on a daily basis. Live in the moment in the best way that you can and don't let anything slip past you or it is gone forever. Appreciate the joy and happiness in your life daily, let the past and the future enhance your life not distract you from it.

My approach to weight loss coaching incorporates these principles in my step by step process. Follow the steps as you would if you were in a coaching relationship. You may not have a coach to talk to in this process but use the book as your support. Keep a journal for getting your thoughts out of your head. That way it makes room for more and it gets your problems out in front of you. This makes it easier to find solutions. If you ask the right questions you will find the right answers.

Complete the tasks that are laid out in this book. They will only take a little time but it is time invested in the rest of your life. Give this new way of losing weight a chance. You might have expected immediate results when losing weight in the past, but now you are trying something new, something different. It is not a diet! It is a mind and a lifestyle change. The results *will* come if you give it a chance to work.

Making these changes now will bring you to a place where you never have to be thinking or obsessing about your weight again. All that space in your mind that was clogged with guilt, anger, shame, points and calories will be free so you can focus on all the wonderful things in your life and give them the attention that they deserve, and live a life of happiness that comes with achieving your goals and realising your dreams.

Are you still holding onto your new thought, "I CAN do this"?

If it has drifted away, or been replaced by anything else, grab it! Bring it back! If you use this book as it is intended, this thought will turn into a belief. It will not only help you to achieve your weight loss dreams but any other dream you have in life too.

Let's take the first step.

Section 2:

The 7 Steps

Chapter 7:

Step 1: How Fed Up am I?

"In order to change,
we must be sick and tired
of being sick and tired"

Author Unknown

This is the all important first question. If you are not motivated enough now to make a change in your life, chances are you won't see this through to the end. It is important at this stage to feel that there is no going back. Are you feeling so Fed Up that the only alternative is to try something new and make a lasting change? Are you fed up of being Fed Up?

Whatever you tried before has not worked, that is why you are here now. There are reasons why the things you tried failed and through the course of this book you will discover what they are and how to get past them in the future. The key is not to let the past failures affect your level of motivation now. If you have ever watched a toddler try something new, they inevitably will fail many times but they don't let these failures stop them from trying again and again. They persevere until they find the right way!

To take that all important step forward you need to be ready and willing to leave the place where you are and never return again. Pain is what drives you to change; you want to move away from it. You need to know it is there and acknowledge it.

So think about how you are feeling right now because of your weight. With the help of Task 1, spend some time thinking about these feelings. Take some time asking yourself these questions. Be honest with yourself.

Now is your time. You have tried many ways before and they didn't work. Make this the last time you will ever spend time, emotions, tears and money on losing weight. Now is YOUR time to change and be the person you want to be. Give it the time it deserves. The time you deserve. Nobody else is ever going to do this for you.

Face the facts, you are the person responsible for where you are now; but you are also the person that can take you to where you want to be.

For change to happen successfully it has to be a MUST, so make it a must for you.

Write your answers in your journal

TASK ONE: *NAME MY EMOTIONS*

- When I look in the mirror what do I see?
- How do I feel when I look in the mirror?
- How is my weight affecting my health? How does this make me feel?
- When I think about how my weight and my health effects my relationships with my partner, my children, my friends, how do I feel?
- How do I feel in social circumstances because of my weight and how I look?
- How confident do I feel every day?
- What will my life be like in 5 or 10 years if I don't change?
- How will I feel if I stay like this?

What kind of emotions did you come up with? Make a list of the feelings.

What do they feel like? Describe what they feel like, their intensity. What is your body doing? Is your breathing shallow or deep? Is your posture upright or lowered?

Learn to recognise what an emotion feels like. Far too often we generalise our emotions and we are not truly aware of what we are really feeling. Is it anger or frustration? Is it sadness or self pity? Is it fear or anxiety? Is it guilt or shame?

Later in this process we will address emotions in greater detail and how they are connected to eating, but for now it is important to know what you are feeling in relation to your weight.

What is your unwanted fat causing you to feel about you and your life?

Give your feelings a number, how intense are they on a scale of 1 to 10?

Now ask yourself:

On a scale of 1 to 10, 1 being "not at all" and 10 being "yes, without any doubt",

- How badly do I want to change?

- How motivated do I feel right now to make the necessary changes?

- How motivated do I feel right now, to achieve my goals?

STRATEGY ONE

If at any stage during this process you feel you are losing motivation and the will to keep up with your changes, return to this page in your journal.

Feel the emotions you describe here.
Remind yourself: "This is how I feel when I am fat".

"I don't want to feel like this anymore"

I have drawn up a sample page of what your journal might look like in case you are unclear about how to start it.

Step 1: My journey to the new me: How fed up am I?

- When I look in the mirror I see a fat woman. I see a large belly, fat dimpled thighs and flabby arms,
- I feel disgusted, depressed, ugly,
- I feel tired all the time, I have no energy, I don't sleep well and I am out of breath walking up the stairs. This upsets me
- I don't feel attractive and sexy so I avoid intimacy with my husband. None of my nice clothes fit me so I don't go out with my husband or my friends. I can't run around with my kids, I get out of breath very quickly.
- I avoid social circumstances, but if I am out, I feel self conscious and awkward
- I don't feel confident at all
- If I don't change now I will be fatter in 10 years, I know my health will suffer, I know weight causes things like high blood pressure, heart disease, diabetes, high cholesterol. I know my life could be cut short if this continues. My marriage could suffer.
- I will become even more depressed and fed up. I won't be happy and I know it will affect me in everything I do. I feel anxious thinking about it

---

My breathing is shallow, my head is down and my posture is slumped. I am feeling depressed and anxious

---

depression is a 9
anxiety is a 10

My motivation to change is a 10   I must change

This is merely an illustration of how to use your journal. You can do it in any way you wish; all I ask is that you answer the questions with complete honesty. You might come up with some answers that are upsetting and painful: this is normal. The truth can hurt sometimes. This is what it takes however, to see things as they are; no better and no worse. When you can see the real picture for what it really is, you will achieve a level of clarity that will help you to move forward.

Don't judge, blame, ridicule or get angry with yourself. There is nothing to be gained. What is done is done. Later, you will learn how to use the past to your benefit. For now, focus on things as they are, as truthfully as you can. Nobody else has to see this journal. It is just for you. You are the one that will benefit greatly from what you write, provided you give it time and effort. After all this is all about you; your time for yourself. Don't you deserve it?

So! How did you do?
- How did you score the level of intensity of your emotions?
- How did you score your motivation to make a change?

If you scored yourself at 7 or above then you are ready to change and ready to put in the effort required.

There is no magic wand or instant pill that is going to lose the weight for you. It is all down to you, with help from me. Fat is not going to disappear without work, but the great thing about the I *CAN* way is that you are creating the lifestyle that can work for you. Once you achieve your weight loss goal, you will be able to maintain it and never again have to feel as you do now.

So far you have established how Fed Up you are being fat. You have also confirmed how badly you want to change.

Keep thinking "I CAN do this"

Now for step 2: it is time to set your goal.

Chapter 8:

Step 2: Setting my Goal

"A goal is a dream with a deadline"

Napoleon Hill

While it is good to have clear and specific goals, they are doomed to fail if they are not realistic and achievable. If a hippo sets his goal to becoming a giraffe, it doesn't matter how hard he tries it's not going to happen.

At this point I would like to reiterate what I said at the beginning of this book when I spoke about what I meant by Fat and what being happy with your body shape is all about. In my dictionary fat is a feeling, not a label or a judgement. If you are feeling fat and it is affecting your life and your happiness, it is time to change it. Just as fat is not about what anyone else thinks, the shape you aspire to be is not about what anyone else thinks either. It is about what will make you happy in yourself.

Don't let our image-obsessed culture, influence you in making unrealistic choices. I urge you to let nothing other than your health affect your decision. Achieving a healthy body as well as a healthy mind is intrinsically part of the process of permanent natural weight loss process. There are guideline measurements available, as I will describe a little later, to help you decide what is considered healthy for your height. But they are merely guidelines and need to be treated as such. They are useful if you have always been overweight and are not sure what a realistic goal would be for you.

For those that have not always been overweight, using your clothes can be a very effective way of setting your goal.

Similarly to what I did when I was setting my goal, many of my clients find they have a pair of jeans that fit them a couple of years before, at a time when they were very happy with their weight. It is specific, it is a clothes size. It is achievable and realistic! They were this size before (without taking extreme measures) and it is compelling; it is associated with a time that they were really happy with their body shape. Don't worry if the item of clothing is no longer in fashion, you don't have to wear it in public, just use it as your tool of measurement!

Using clothes as a guide of measurement is also especially useful if you have been easily put off in the past by the number on the weighing scales. Your clothes will never lie. If they are feeling looser, then your body shape is changing.

The scales can be so easily influenced so easily by many factors:

- Excess salt leads to fluid retention, the sodium in your body holds onto more water. *Result: the scales are not a true reflection of your weight.*
- Not drinking enough water, your body holds onto the water it has as it doesn't know when more will be coming. *Result: the scales are not a true reflection of your weight.*
- Stress; stress hormones can cause water retention. *Result: the scales are not a true reflection of your weight.*
- Hormonal changes, e.g. PMS, these changes can cause your body to retain more water. *Result: the scales are not a true reflection of your weight.*

If you are someone that can be thrown off by your weight fluctuating in the wrong direction, then change your focus. Don't focus on the number on weighing scales; use your clothes as a guide. Throw away the scales. They will not help you.

This is the time for positive good things in your life; there is only room for what will help you to make the progress you want. There are a number of guides you can use to get an idea of what size is healthy for you.

> The BMI scale uses your height, in relation to your weight and categorises you as, "Underweight", "Healthy", Overweight", "Obese", or "Very Obese".

> There is a school of thought this is not a good guide as muscle weighs more than fat, therefore rendering it inaccurate. This is a fair point, but let's face it: you know yourself if you are carrying more fat or more muscle. If it is fat you are carrying then it is a good guide to what range you are in.

> Bear in mind that this is just a guide, combine it with the point at which you feel healthy and happy.

There are other guides available for measuring your size in relation to your health. One of these is to calculate your waist to hip ratio. With a measuring tape you can measure you waist. To find your waist, with your finger find the top of your hips and the bottom of your ribs, your waist is in between these two points. Then measure your hips at their widest point. Divide your hip measurement into your waist measurement.

> So for example your waist is 34 inches and your hips are 36 inches. 34/36 = 0.94

If you are a woman this measurement puts you in the high risk category for such diseases as high blood pressure, diabetes and coronary heart disease. If you are a man then you are at lower risk of these diseases. A woman ideally should be 0.80 or less and a man should be 0.95 or less.

I find these two methods are the best guides that are available for helping you to clarify what is healthy for you and in turn, helping you to set your goal.

A SMART Goal

The SMART model is widely used for setting goals:

Specific – What is it you really want to achieve?
Measurable – How can you measure your progress?
Appealing – How compelling and inspiring is your goal?
Realistic – Is this goal something that is achievable?
Timed- When is your deadline for this goal to be achieved?

How do I get there?

"It is not enough to take steps
which may lead to a goal:
Each step must be itself
a goal and a step likewise"

Johann Wolfgang Von Goethe

Once you have decided on your main goal it is important to decide on each step you are going to take to achieve it. This is a wonderful way of working towards any goal you set in any area of your life. Setting and achieving a goal is like climbing a mountain. It takes work, perseverance and the *I CAN attitude*: but the rewards are exhilarating.

This is something that became very clear to me when I climbed Ben Nevis, the highest mountain in the United Kingdom, in 2009. I climbed it with my husband who carried our eight month old on his back! It was only the third mountain I had tackled and I found it extremely challenging. I very nearly did not make it; there was a point when I was ready to give up. I hit a very big metaphorical wall.

I sat down to ask myself if I had what it took to continue, when a man passing me said "You are nearly there, it's worth the pain to get to the top!" I realised then how badly I did want to get to the top and from somewhere deep inside I found the energy, drive and determination to take the last steps to achieving my goal.

The view from the summit was spectacular. I felt exhilaration like I had never felt before. Mental and physical pain and exhaustion were instantly dissipated as I looked out on one of most breathtaking views I had ever seen. I had challenged myself to my extremes and I had succeeded in achieving my goal. Overcoming physical and psychological obstacles, I achieved what I had set out to do. I faced the point of submitting to my self-limiting beliefs and giving up, but I chose to continue.

This is the greatest metaphor I can use to describe the journey to achieving goals.
Climbing a mountain and achieving goals, are comparable in many ways:

- You must believe you can do it.
- You will only get there by taking one step at a time.
- You will face obstacles along the way that you must overcome to carry on.
- One slip does not mean you are back where you started.
- If you focus completely on the top of the mountain or on your final goal you will miss out on the beauty that surrounds you along the way, it is as much about the journey as it is about the destination.
- The feelings of joy, achievement and exhilaration when you reach the top or your goal are truly amazing.

Fat and Fed Up, No More!
7 Steps to Permanent Natural Weight Loss

Breaking a goal down into smaller steps makes it more manageable and less daunting. It also helps you to monitor your progress, as you can see clearly what you are achieving. In my situation I had three stone to lose, to bring me back to the size I was when I got married and it was when I was happy with my body shape. I wanted to slip into a pair of sleek, black trousers I wore for work. Getting back into them was achieving the goal!

I knew by doing this the healthy natural way it was going to take some time, because the healthy way to lose weight was 1 or 2 lbs a week. So being realistic to lose 42 lbs it was going to take between 6 and 7 months. I gave myself 7 months. That's a daunting and off putting length of time. I chose to break it down.

In the past I was obsessed with scales, I used to weigh myself every day, sometimes a couple of times a day. I decided it was time I stopped letting the scales dictate how I was going to feel. If I was up in pounds I could be fed up for the day and beat myself up over it.

That was the old me: now I use my clothes as my guide. I purposely picked out 3 pairs of trousers that were different sizes. I always chose trousers as they were a good indicator of the size of your waist, hips, bum and thighs. If any of these were getting smaller your trousers will tell you. I tried on the largest and wrote down how it felt, i.e., tight on the waist and hips, difficult to close, ok on the thighs.

I had no idea how long it was going to take to make these feel comfortable. For 3 weeks I followed the plans I had made for myself and when I tried on the trousers again, while holding my breath with anticipation, anxiety, hope and fear, I found that they fitted. In fact they were a little loose.

I was elated! My efforts worked and with relative ease. I had not needed to diet or push myself to any limits. I changed my lifestyle in a healthy and natural way and it had worked. I rewarded myself with an Andrea Bocelli CD.

That is how my step by step approach worked. I moved onto the next slightly smaller pair of trousers and did the same thing. 7 months seem to fly by and by the end of it I had exceeded my goal by losing an extra half a stone.

I had to fill my wardrobe with new clothes that were a size smaller than I had been in a long time. However, this time I had achieved this body shape in a natural healthy way without restricting myself or pushing myself to extremes.

By the time the 7 months had passed, my new way of thinking and living was automatic and natural and I have not looked back since. It is now my normal way of living.

Now it is your turn. Complete task 2 in your journal.

Using the SMART model now decide on and write down your goal. Then break this goal into smaller more manageable steps, give them a time limit and implement a rewards system for achieving each step.

TASK TWO: *SETTING MY GOAL*

- What is my goal?
  (Make it very specific and clear)

- Is this goal realistic and achievable for me?

- How happy will I be when I achieve this goal?
- What does achieving this goal mean to me?
- How will achieving my goal change my life for the better?

- When do I want to have achieved this goal?
  Is it short term (3 months)
  Is it medium term (4 months to a year)
  Is it long term (longer than 1 year)

- What could stop me from achieving my goal?
  How will I overcome these obstacles?

- What small steps am I going to take to achieve my goal?
- When I am going to have achieved each step?
- How am I going to measure my progress?
- What reward am I going to give myself for achieving each step?

- How will I reward myself when I achieve my goal?

Goal Mountain

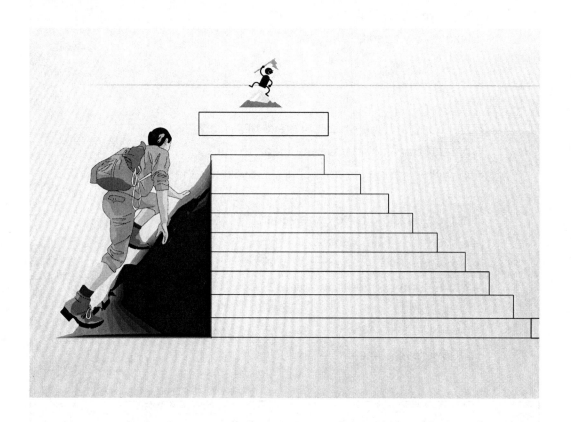

Use Goal Mountain to help you to realise your dreams: Fill in your goal at the top, then write in each space provided what steps you are going to take to achieve this goal.

Refer to it on a regular basis and as you achieve each step tick it off.

This will allow you to see what progress you are making and it also evokes the feeling of achievement as you cross off your smaller goals as you are going along. Our achievements, no matter how small they seem should always be acknowledged and rewarded. Don't take anything that you achieve for granted.

So far in this process, you have identified how you feel as you are now, in the body shape you are in. You know what these emotions are and how they make you feel. You have decided you have had enough. It is time for change. It is time to move forward to the place you want to be.

Next you identified what you want the future to look like. The future you want for yourself. You decided on your goal. You know what it is you want and you are now going to focus on it and achieve it.

Are you still thinking "I CAN do this"?

When you are thinking these words then you are focusing on what you CAN do and CAN achieve. There is only one way to do this. You have tried dieting before and it didn't work. It is time for something new, it is time for the I CAN way and there is no other way. No other way to achieve your success. Think I CAN, Focus on I CAN, Do I CAN and in time you will Believe I CAN and nothing will stop you from achieving your goals and realising your dreams.

Now let's take a brief look back so it can help you to move forward, take Step 3.

STRATEGY TWO

Whatever it is you want in life write it down, be clear and specific and set yourself a deadline when you want to have achieved it.

Break it down into smaller steps if you need to. It brings more clarity and it helps you to monitor your progress.

You CAN get whatever it is you desire, if you are clear about what it is you want.

Chapter 9:

Step 3: What Can I Learn from the Past?

"To look backward for a while is to refresh the eye,
to restore it and to render it more fit
for its prime function of looking forward"

Margaret Fairless Barber

Part of what Coaching helps you to do is to learn new tools and strategies to help you on your journey to achieving your goals and realising your dreams. It helps you to move forward. Before we take the next step on your journey to achieving your goal, I encourage you to spend some time putting together the lessons that are waiting to be learned from the past. Your successes and your failures from the past can show you what works and what doesn't work for you when trying to lose weight.

Know Your Habits and Patterns

At this stage it is important to identify why you are here. What have you been doing that has caused you to feel fat? What habits and patterns have you developed over the years that are responsible for your excess weight? This entire process is about you being honest with yourself so that you can see things as they really are. This book however is not about giving you a label or putting you in a category of eater, i.e., compulsive eater, binge eater, comfort eater etc. I don't believe in categorising or pigeon holing people. The facts are the facts. What are you doing that is making you put on weight? No one is force feeding you. You are putting the food in your mouth. You are responsible for where you are now.

Don't get me wrong I don't want you blaming yourself or beating yourself up about what you have been doing. Bin your judgements right now.

This is an exercise to help you see things as they are, be honest with yourself. You need clarity. It is very easy to generalise what is going on or to see things with rose tinted glasses.

One of my clients told me she could not understand how she was putting on weight. She was getting fatter but she walked most days and her diet was pretty healthy. She listed off the food she would eat for her 3 meals and yes, they were healthy.

This is the general description. When we got to the specifics of her day we discovered that her portion sizes were actually enough for 2 people, she thought it was normal.

She also would sit in front of the television in the evenings and eat sweet things. She was doing it so unconsciously that she was not even aware of how much she was eating. She would turn on the television and take out a box of biscuits or sweets and graze away all evening. Straight away after this exercise she could see the behaviour that was causing her weight gain. When I asked her to write down over the course of the week exactly what she would eat and how much, she was shocked. Now she could see things clearly. She could see her behaviour as it was and why she was fat.

So at this stage don't think about why you are engaging in certain behaviours, we will look at this later. You are taking one step at a time. For now identify what you are doing, what you are eating. It is about bringing everything you are doing into your consciousness, being aware. Describe, don't judge. This task will help you to identify your patterns and habits. When you know they are there, they won't be able to sneak up and and ambush you later.

TASK THREE: *KNOW MY HABITS*

Think about the last week/month in your life. What are your patterns?

- What do you eat for breakfast? If any.
- How much do you eat?
- What do you eat between breakfast and lunch?
- How much do you eat?
- What do you eat for lunch? If any
- How much do you eat
- What do you eat between lunch and dinner?
- How much do you eat?
- What do you eat for dinner? If any
- How much do you eat?
- What do you eat after dinner?
- How much do you eat?
- What do you eat before you go to bed?
- How much do you eat?
- Are there times of the day that you eat when you are not hungry?
- What makes you eat when you are not hungry?
- Are there times you eat and you don't realise you are eating?
- How much do you eat?
- Do you get up in the night to eat?
- How much do you eat?

Remember be honest. The only person you are trying to fool is yourself and that won't help you achieve your goal.

Make a list of the habits and patterns that you can identify.

STRATEGY THREE

When you know what your habits and patterns are, you are not at the mercy of them anymore. They cannot unconsciously destroy what you want in life. Identify them.

Write them down. Make a list.

When you know they are there you can then work on where they came from and how you can change them to work best for you.

Now that you have identified the behaviour that has made you fat, we will learn from what you have tried in the past to lose it.

The Past and the Lessons it holds

The past can be the very thing to stop you from being able to think and believe "I CAN". If you have tried something in the past and have failed to achieve your desired result, then it is an automatic conclusion that all these failures mean it can't be done. It might be an automatic conclusion to draw but it is NOT accurate. All that is true is the WAY didn't work.

When it comes to losing weight the first thing most of us turn to are diets, supplements and meal replacement products. We restrict ourselves on a daily basis, we eat what someone else says we should and when they say we should. We force ourselves into strict exercise regimes that someone else decides for us.

We count the calorie content of our food and live each day wondering "have we burned off enough to lose a pound?" When a time comes that we break out of this strict regime and eat something that is not allowed we feel all is lost and revert back to what we did before we started the diet. We gain any weight we might have lost and end up feeling more frustrated and disappointed and fed up.

It is not surprising that this way of losing weight does not work. It is a completely unhealthy means to losing weight. It goes against everything natural in your body and disconnects you completely from it. We will look at this in more detail a little later but the important thing to remember at this stage is that you are not a failure; you failed to achieve your goal because the means you used were not practical. You cannot beat yourself up for that. You CAN lose weight; it is just time to do it in a different way. Your past experiences are not a waste, however; you can learn from what you did in the past.

No matter what you do in life, whether it is something great or a great mistake, if you can take some learning or wisdom from it, then its value has no limit. By looking at the past you can gain huge insight into how to live your life in the present and how you can live in the future.

You can see how you reacted to certain situations, what you did when you did something well and when you did something badly. By taking the time to look back you can gain so much that will help you now and in the future.

When I say looking back however I only recommend it to facilitate learning lessons and insights. There is a difference between this and living in the past. If you spend your time overly attached to the past or a specific incident that occurred there you will have no time left to look forward to the future or time to live in your present.

I want to emphasise some important points here. If there is something in the past that you feel you cannot get past or leave behind, it might be useful to see a qualified Counsellor or Therapist.

They can help you to work through the experience and how it has impacted on you, so that you can make sense of it and move forward. Sometimes an experience that has caused us trauma or pain, emotionally or physically, can hinder us from moving forward. It can be difficult to work through it on our own.

Often we spend many years suffering because of an experience. It might take help from a professional-
- but when you can see that you are more than your experience:
- more than what happened to you - and that nothing can destroy you unless you let it;
- you can begin to move away from the past and leave it where it belongs.

Looking back is especially useful when you are facing a new challenge in your life and you are in doubt about your ability to overcome it. Chances are, in your past you have faced other challenges, some that you may have forgotten about, some that were huge at the time, but might not seem so significant now. The methods that you used to overcome these challenges can be used and/or adapted to help you over the current obstacle. Similarly, if you failed to meet a challenge and failed to succeed then there is a lesson there also.

Along with remembering the methods you used in the past to deal with a situation, it is hugely important to acknowledge the strength, courage, persistence, self belief, determination, etc, that you may have used. If you have used them before you can be sure you can find them again.

In Step 4 we will look at how the past may have led you to develop certain beliefs that impact on the way you live your life now, but for the moment we will focus on the lessons that can be learned from your actions specifically in relation to what you did to lose weight and exercise.

Some things belong in the past - Dieting

From my personal and professional experience diets don't work. Not in the long term. Would you agree with me? How many have you tried? I have lost count of how many I have tried over the years. When I talk about diets I mean anything that goes against the natural way of eating. It can be following a restrictive plan that someone else develops or it can be restricting yourself on your own.

I started becoming obsessed about my weight when I was about 16. I took to eating very little. I would pretend to whomever I was with that I wasn't very hungry or that I had already eaten. You become a very good liar when it comes to controlling your food intake. It can take the form of hiding the large amount of food you eat or lying about how little you eat.

I continued this way throughout my years in College. Ironically in college, Susie Orbach's book, Fat is a Feminist Issue, was part of my Sociology syllabus. Despite this book being a hugely insightful look at how we can turn food into a friend and find ways to accept ourselves as we are and not fall prey to how society depicts how a woman should look, it never impacted on me. It was the wrong time for me. I was so caught up in being thin. That was what I wanted. I was not concerned with what made people fat and relationships people had with food. I only cared about how I looked. My happiness was down to how thin I was that was what I believed. I was not ready or open to change.

Restriction is the reason why diets don't work. We enter into a psychology of denial. We deny ourselves everyday and instead of this working in our favour we focus so much on what we can't have, it becomes all we want. Invariably what we cut out of our lives so dramatically is what we will binge on after dieting.

When following a diet we are also doing what someone else is telling us to do. Someone else is telling us what to eat, what not to eat and when to eat it.

This invariably leads us to feeling hungry most of the time. If we don't listen to our bodies how do we know what it is our own body actually needs?

We don't. We give up the ability to connect with our bodies and in turn we lose trust in what our body knows and is trying to tell us. I believe if we connected with, listened to and trusted in our bodies we would never be fat. You will learn how to do this later in the book in Step 5.

It is so important for us to understand why something doesn't work. This will help us to avoid repeating the ridiculous strategies of diets, which only serve to make the diet industry richer and ourselves fatter. Not only is it important to understand why diets don't work in general, it is so important that you understand why they didn't work for you.

- What is it about the different diets that you tried that led you straight back to where you started?
- Why could you not sustain any weight loss?
- How long did it take for you to stop the diet?
- What caused you to stop?

Diets: learn from them but leave them in the past.

Specifically in relation to weight loss, by looking to your past you will learn so much. For example -

1. You will know what you have tried.
2. You will know what worked and for how long.
3. You will see what didn't work.
4. You can see how much money you have spent in the past trying to lose weight.
5. You will see why a particular diet may have worked for a while.
6. You will see why a particular diet failed.
7. You will see how you reacted to the diets and what you did to sabotage them and what they did to sabotage you.

Exercising: What did I do in the past? What can I learn?

To know what you are going to do in the future to bring the right movement into your life, have a look at what you tried before and how it worked or didn't work for you. Did you join numerous gyms for a year and use your membership for about 2 months? Did you buy exercise DVDs every other week and hardly ever use them? Did you go walking but decide once the winter came that it was too dark and the weather too bad to maintain it?

There are two main reasons for giving up on exercise:

1. We choose the wrong one for our lifestyle: what we choose to do turns out to be very difficult to maintain due to work and family commitments. So we focus on why we can't do it instead of looking at what we CAN factor into our lifestyles easily. After a while we stop

and say, "I tried but I just don't have the time"

2. Our attitudes to exercising. Many of us say regularly, "I hate exercise", "Exercise is so boring", "I get nothing out of exercising"

The purpose of the task within this chapter is to show you how there is something to be learned from everything. The diets did not work for different reasons but by identifying these reasons they will in turn serve as a tool for moving you away from the place you have been. The time when you went from one failed diet to another and could never really work out why nothing was working.

You can also learn why you have failed to maintain some movement in your life. You can identify what your biggest blocks are in relation to moving right. Then you can use this awareness to create your new movement that will fit into your life in a way that you can sustain.

TASK THREE part 2: *WHAT CAN I LEARN FROM MY PAST?*

Make a list of all the diets you have used in the past.

Make a list of all the things you did not like about each of these diets.

Write down why you think these diets did not work for you.

Make a list of any positive things you learned – such as healthy tasty recipes.

Of these positives things you learned which could you use in the future as part of your new healthy lifestyle? For example, new healthy options for meals

PART B:

Make a list of all the exercise routines/plans you had in the past.

Make a list of the things that stopped you maintaining them.

Make a list of the things you liked about these plans.

What insights about exercise can you take from all of this that will help you in the future? What do you need to avoid or make happen?

> *Now have you a list of all the things that you need to avoid in the future when it comes to eating right and moving right? Also have you a list of what you CAN use and what CAN work for you in the future?*

STRATEGY THREE part 2

If you are ever faced with something in life that you feel you cannot handle, take some time to look to your past to see if you ever faced something similar before.

- *What did you do?*
- *Did it work?*
- *What could you have done differently?*
- *What skills and attributes did it require?*
- *Do you still have them?*

You think you don't have what it takes to deal with it –

- *What does it take to deal with a situation?*
- *Have you ever used these at any time in the past?*
- *What have you learned from your past that might help you?*

Never let the past be a waste. There is much to learn from hindsight. If you learn something from what you have done before, good or bad, its value is infinite.

The Secret to Weight loss Success

I believe there are three things we need to do to lose weight and to keep it off. When all three are done together we can achieve whatever weight loss goal we have and maintain it for life.

Have you ever wondered why you always end up back in the same place, no matter what diet you try and no matter how much exercise you do? You stick to the rigid eating plan and force yourself to run 5ks a day and while you manage to lose the weight initially, it always creeps back on.

Have you envied people who appear to lose weight effortlessly and manage to keep it off?

The reason why you have not managed to maintain your weight loss is because you have not been doing the three things that are necessary for long term weight loss success. The people that seem to lose weight effortlessly are making the same effort, but they are also doing the three things together.

Are you ready to learn the Secret to Permanent Weight Loss?

The Weight Loss Triad

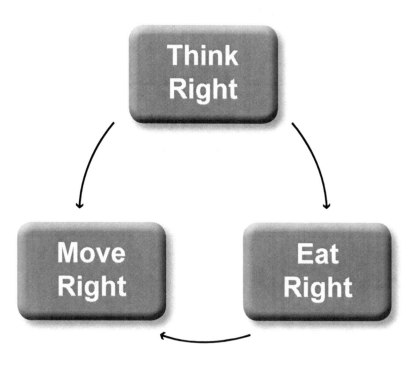

Are you ready to change the way in which you want to lose weight?

Do you want this to be the last time you ever have to lose weight?

Do you want to learn how to lose weight and keep it off for life?

You are? Then make the Weight Loss Triad part of your new lifestyle every day and achieve your goal and realise your dreams.

My clients say to me all the time, "If I didn't learn to *Think Right* first I would never have been able to *Move Right* and *Eat Right*". This is a very good point and the reason that most diets fail. Without working on what is going on in your head in relation to food and your body, then any attempts to lose weight are not going to last: because your own mind will sabotage your efforts in time and it will go back to doing what you have allowed it to do for so many years.

"The state of your life is nothing more than a reflection of the state of your mind"

Wayne Dyer

So let's start with your mind.

Chapter 10:

Step 4: Think Right!

> **"If you don't like something, change it.
> If you can't change it,
> change the way you think about it."**
>
> *Mary Engolbreit*

The *Think Right* part of the Weight Loss Triad involves working on your mind, giving your head the work out it deserves. Later, we will work on your eating plan, you will learn techniques for controlling your portions and you will also develop a movement plan that is right for you. However, without working on your mind first these new plans are doomed to fail.

What you focus on is what you get

Focusing is a huge part of thinking right. Focusing means to aim your attention at, to home in on and to concentrate on something specific. Basically what you focus on is what you get. Have you ever observed other people who always seem to be negative and pessimistic? Very often more and more negative things happen to them. Or so it seems. Do bad things always happen to them or is it the way they perceive a situation? On the other hand, those people that always seem to be positive and optimistic, good things always happen to them. Or so it seems!

People who automatically see the negative side of life are always going to see the worst in a situation first. Alternatively for those who are more on the positive side, they will make the best of a situation.

It depends on what they choose to focus on.

Some examples of these types:

Negative:
"It is lashing with rain outside, now I can't take the kids on a picnic like I planned. The day is ruined."

Positive:
"It is lashing with rain outside, we can't do the picnic but, we can go for a walk. The kids will have great fun in their rain coats and wellingtons splashing in the puddles."

Negative:
"I lost my job. I only have a bit of money to keep me going for a short while. There are no jobs out there. It is terrible."

Positive:
"I lost my job. I have a bit of money to keep me going for a short while so I am ok in the immediate future. I can use this opportunity to look for something new to do. I was getting tired of my old job. It's time for new beginnings."

Negative:
"I have tried so many diets and none of them has worked. I am never going to lose weight, I will always be fat."

Positive:
"I have tried so many diets and none of them worked for me. If I am going to lose weight I will have to try something new. The old ways don't work. I will look for a new way."

No matter what the issue is, positive or negative thinking is all about the focus you choose to apply to the situation.

Whether you succeed or fail at anything in life it is going to depend on what you focus on, because you will either be focused on what you CAN do or what you CAN'T. Focusing on I CAN helps you find solutions, focusing on I CAN'T means you only see the problems.

What you focus on is what you feel

What you are focusing on is also going to impact on your emotional state. If you are focusing on the negative you are not going to be feeling happy. If you are thinking about something happy you are not going to be feeling sad. At the beginning of this process you identified how fed up you were. This was vital to push you forward. Now, however, it is time to change your focus from being fed up.

If you are focusing on how fed up you are, you are going to be feeling it too. Now it is time to focus on how you are going to feel when you achieve your goal and how you are feeling now that you are doing something to change your situation.

This requires positive focus and positive language - *I CAN do this*. When you are feeling positive emotions your body reacts in a specific way. Your posture is more upright, your breathing is deeper and you are more relaxed.

You are more in control! Have you noticed this before?

Try it right now, think of a time or a situation when you were really happy, see yourself there at that time, what were you doing? Who was there? What were you saying? What were you thinking? What was your body doing? How is your body now just remembering this situation?

Are you feeling happy just remembering it? If you really put yourself back into this memory you will be feeling happy just from thinking about it.

To contrast this, let's go back to the first task I gave you. I asked you to identify the emotions you were feeling because of your body shape. I asked you to name each of them and to describe how you were feeling and how your body felt. Do you remember? Look back to your journal to see what you wrote. At this stage you were focusing on how unhappy you were. Your language was negative and your posture was reflecting this negativity.

Anthony Robbins, the American peak performance coach, believes that these three forces, 1) focus, 2) language and 3) physiology, are interconnected parts of your emotional state, but they are also things that can be controlled and changed by you. Can you see how you were able to feel happy just by focusing on a happy memory, by thinking about something that made you feel good? This is a powerful technique that will help you in this process and in any area of your life.

Have you ever had one of those days where you felt everything was going wrong and you wished you never got out of bed? You might have wakened up tired and off form. Something happens early in the day, something small, burnt toast, dropped cereal, the dog yelping. Whatever it was it put you in a worse mood. Then something else happens, you end up late for work, or you forget your lunch or your pens keep running out. Nothing that is absolutely terrible happens but it all joins forces to make you feel more frustrated and annoyed over the course of the day.

It seems like everything is going wrong. It *seems* like it; however, everything is not going wrong. It is just a few little things that happened but because of your emotional state it feels much worse than what it is. Every day, something small like this can happen, but if you are feeling upbeat and happy you don't even notice it.

A negative state is not going to help you to have a good day or help you to achieve your goals. The next time you wake up feeling off form or feeling down and lacking in the drive and desire to continue with your goal, identify what you are feeling.

What emotions are there? What are you focusing on? What language are your thoughts using? Is it negative, disempowering, self defeating? What is your body doing? Identify and acknowledge what is going on - and then change it. Change your focus, your language and your physiology together. Use the memory technique to bring you to a positive, happy time or choose to focus on the positive side of the situation, pushing out the negative thoughts. When you learn how to do this with ease, which will only come with practice and repetition, you can get yourself out of an emotional state that is not helping you and go to one which is going to help you to achieve your goals.

In Step One, you admitted how you feel because of your weight and your body shape. In Step Two, you decided on your goal. You chose what it is you want for you. It is time to move on. Your goal is the place you want to move to. You identified how you are going to feel when you achieve it. Focus on these feelings, these new positive happy feelings. Focus on the new you that is emerging, and how good it makes you feel. This focus will in turn give you the energy to achieve what it is you need to do to get to your goal.

At this point we need to clarify something: there is a distinct difference between focus and obsession. When you are obsessed with something you are consumed by it, you are infatuated with it; you eat, breathe and sleep it. Possibly you have been like this in the past with your weight. Thoughts of food, eating it or not eating it, the amount of calories you have eaten or burned, consume your entire mind. Your whole day from your waking moment might have been devoted to thinking about losing weight. *This is an obsession*. It is time to stop obsessing about losing weight and instead focus on what it is you want and focus on the steps you need to take to achieve it.

Understanding your world

"Men are disturbed not by events,
but by the views which they take of them"

Epictetus AD 55 – AD 135

Knowing what you want and concentrating on it are so important in achieving a goal, but unfortunately no matter how hard we can try to do this we can actually sabotage ourselves from getting the results we want. It's true, no matter how badly you want something you can actually stop yourself from getting it.

Have you ever wondered why it is so difficult to maintain weight loss during and after a diet? Outside of the psychology of denial that we identified earlier, diets don't work because they don't help us to work on what is going on in our minds. What goes on in our minds, whether we are aware of it or not, is ultimately responsible for our emotions, our behaviours and our actions and ultimately the results we get, such as a fat body.

Our beliefs are what go on in our minds. Beliefs are a set of principles that we have, often since childhood, that guide our thoughts, our emotions and our actions. They are responsible for how we see the world and reality. These can be good and rational beliefs that help you to achieve happiness and fulfilment or they can be limiting and self defeating and serve as the biggest obstacle to achieving your success.

According to American psychologist Albert Ellis the founder of Rational Emotive Behaviour Therapy, changing self limiting or self defeating beliefs is the key to resolving problems and becoming healthy.

He believed and showed that beliefs determine the way human beings feel and behave. He believed that the reactions we have to having our goals blocked or even thinking they might be blocked is determined by what we believe to be true. To illustrate this he developed a simple format he called the "ABC" Model.

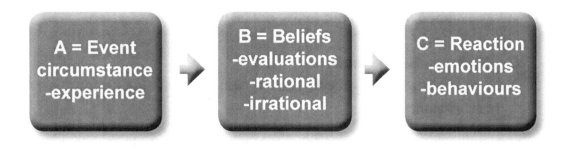

Source: Counselling Resource Website: www.counsellingresource.com

"A" - is the event or the experience or the circumstance, something happens

"B" - are the thoughts or beliefs you have about that experience, they can be rational or irrational

"C"- is the reaction, the feelings you have and the behaviours you carry out because of B

Examples of this:

A. **What happens:**
You weigh yourself and you are 3 pounds heavier than last week.

B. **What you Believe about A:**
You believe that if you gain a pound or two you might never stop gaining weight.

C. **Your Reaction to B:**
You feel extremely unhappy and depressed and go on a strict diet.

A. **What Happens:**
You cook a meal for your family but all the food is not eaten.

B. **What you Believe about A:**
You believe that food should not be wasted under any circumstances.

C. **Your Reaction to B:**
You feel anxious that there is food on the plates and that it will be wasted, so you finish every bit of food on the table.

These examples show it is not actually the event itself that cause the behaviour it is in fact the reaction to the belief about the event. Self defeating or irrational beliefs are described as such because of what they do:

- They can distort our reality; we can evaluate situations, people and the world in an illogical way.
- They stop us from achieving our goals.
- They can cause us to experience extreme emotions which can be distressing and paralysing.

- They can cause behaviours that may lead us to harming ourselves or others.

What we think and tell ourselves in different situations depends on our core beliefs or our set of rules. These can be also rational or irrational. These core beliefs are what determine how we react to life situations. When an event happens it triggers a set of thoughts that are dependent on the subconscious set of rules we have.

To illustrate this I will use the examples from above:

A. **What happens:**
   You weigh yourself and you are 3 pounds heavier than last week.

B. **What you Believe about A:**
   You believe that if you gain a pound or two you might never stop gaining weight.

C. **Your Reaction to B:**
   You feel extremely unhappy and depressed and go on a strict diet.

The Core Belief:
I need to maintain very strict control over my body.

A. **What Happens:**
   You cook a meal for all the family but all the food is not eaten.

B. **What you Believe about A:**
   You believe that food should not be wasted under any circumstances.

C. **Your Reaction to B:**
   You feel anxious that there is food on the plates and that it will be

wasted, so you finish every bit of food on the table.

The Core Belief:
Being wasteful is a sin.

The important thing to remember is that these limiting and self defeating beliefs, which keep you stuck in life, can be challenged and changed. Rational beliefs are based in realistic thinking. Thinking that is based on facts and reality as opposed to subjective opinions or wishful thinking.

Again I will use the examples from above to illustrate rational thinking.

A. **What happens:**
You weigh yourself and you are 3 pounds heavier than last week.

B. **What you Believe about A:**
It is ok to gain a pound or two as a weighing scale is influenced by so many things other than fat.

C. **Your Reaction to B:**
You check how your clothes feel on you, you feel comfortable happy and healthy.

Core Belief:
My happiness comes from within.

A. **What Happens:**
You cook a meal for all the family but all the food is not eaten.

B. **What you Believe about A:**
You believe that eating more food than you need is a waste

C. **Your Reaction to B:**
You put the leftovers in the fridge for lunch the next day.

Core Belief:
It is a shame to waste anything if it can be avoided.

Rational thinking is life enhancing. Irrational thinking is not!

- Rational thinking is based on reality; it is about seeing things as they really are and tolerating what comes with it.
- It supports your goals.
- It creates emotions that are healthy and that you can handle.
- It helps to promote healthy behaviours that assist you in life.

You have the power to change your irrational thoughts and beliefs to rational ones. It involves acknowledging them first. Identify them and bring them into your consciousness.

Your task now is to work on identifying your own beliefs. No-one else's beliefs matter, but your own. They are the ones that have been guiding you all along. You identified in task 1, that your weight and body shape cause you to feel a certain way: Fed up.

You have been unable to achieve your goal to date, every diet you have tried has not been successful, because limiting beliefs have held you back and sabotaged your efforts. Become aware of these beliefs now, the beliefs that haven't made you happy. Now it is time to change them, to consciously choose new life-enhancing beliefs that will empower you to become the person you have always wanted.

If you are uncertain about what your beliefs are as they might be locked away in your unconscious for so long, it might take a little bit of extra time to discover what they are.

Identify your Beliefs

There are 2 ways to identify your beliefs. 1) is to start with the behaviour and work backwards. 2) Is to listen to the chatter or the talk in your head. This negative self talk, or the Gremlin as it is named in the coaching world, or the "Monster" as it is described by some of my clients, are your irrational beliefs.

Number 1 involves addressing the behaviour and identifying what is the underlying cause of it. As we learned earlier in this chapter as Ellis identified in his work there is a flow that happens –

   a) An event; then
   b) We internalise it and apply our beliefs whether rational or irrational; and
   c) As a consequence we have a feeling or behaviour or both.

To illustrate:

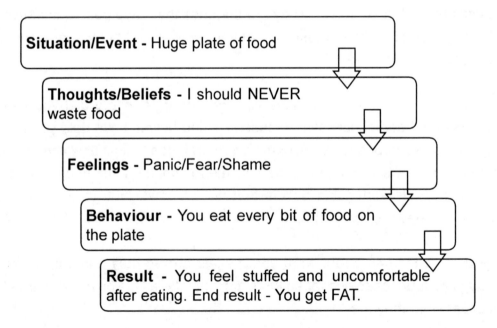

Situation/Event - Huge plate of food

Thoughts/Beliefs - I should NEVER waste food

Feelings - Panic/Fear/Shame

Behaviour - You eat every bit of food on the plate

Result - You feel stuffed and uncomfortable after eating. End result - You get FAT.

If your actions in life are causing you to feel miserable and fed up then the only way to eliminate this is to get to the root cause; that is - your thoughts and beliefs. We will look at negative self talk a little later. In terms of your beliefs if you can't identify them easily then start with the end result. In this example you are feeling stuffed and uncomfortable after every meal.

Ask yourself:

➢ "What has caused me to eat everything on the plate even though I was full?"

➢ "What made me feel panicked and fearful when I thought about leaving some food?"

➢ "How long have I been eating everything on my plate because I felt I had to?"

➢ "What makes me feel so afraid to leave food on my plate?"

➢ "What is wrong with leaving some food on my plate?"

If you ask yourself the right questions you will always find the right answer if you are open to it. Very often we are afraid of the answer so we don't "go there"; we know it might bring some pain. So we avoid it. If you are determined to make a change in your life then facing some pain is sometimes unavoidable. When you see with clarity then you can also see what you need to do: first you must be prepared to accept the answers.

Very often when my clients are in a similar situation to the above they discover that in their childhood they were told it was shameful to waste food, or that it was a sin, that so many children have no food and that it is wrong to waste what is in front of you. Some were not allowed to leave the table until every morsel of food was gone. When this has been your experience in the early years of your life it is not surprising that the thought

---

of wasting food would be one that would cause some panic and fear.

When you are identifying your beliefs and discovering where they came from it is very important to leave judgement in the bin: that's where it belongs. Many criticise themselves for thinking in such ways when they identify their irrational beliefs. I constantly remind people that beliefs are your interpretations of an event that you experienced and that belief was born to help you in that given situation. This is not to be judged or ridiculed. It is what happened! It is what it is!

> The fact of the matter is that this particular belief does not serve a worthwhile purpose now in this stage of your life, so identifying this and making the necessary changes is the path that will take you to your goals and enhance your life.

Don't judge yourself for a decision that you made a long time ago. You made them for specific reasons at the time. It is now time for *new* decisions and *new* beliefs.

The second way to identify your beliefs is to analyse your self talk. Do you ever hear words in your head, such as: I should, I can't, I mustn't, I could never, I need to, I have to.

This negative talk is usually the judgemental and rigid voice. It inhibits you from achieving and moving forward. Its primary aim is to protect you and avoid pain or harm. The fact is: it is rooted in preconceived notions and interpretations of experiences that no longer serve you in a productive way. They are now obsolete but continue to govern your life in a way that is restricting you, stopping you from taking risks and trying new things.

Examples of this chatter include messages like:

- I can't trust my body
- I am too fat

- I should eat now because it is lunch time
- I can't lose weight
- I won't be able to stick to exercise
- I have to clean my plate
- I can't change
- I am too old to change now
- There is no point making changes, they won't last
- I ate too much at the weekend, I have failed
- I can't be bothered
- It won't make any difference
- It never worked before, it won't work now

The key to getting rid of this self defeating chatter is, like your beliefs, to challenge it. Ask the right questions, e.g.

- Why can't I change?
- Who says I am too old to exercise?
- What will happen if I don't clean my plate?
- Why can't I trust my body?
- What's stopping me from losing weight?
- How can I be sure changes won't last?

By acknowledging what is being said in your head and challenging it, you will be able to tune out the unhelpful thoughts and retune yourself to only listen to the thoughts that are truly helping you to achieve your goals.

> You have the right answers within you; it is just a matter of finding them. Listen to your inner voice, take on board the wisdom it has to offer that will benefit you.

Imagine your mind as a garden. You have made the decision to do some gardening, to make your garden a place where you can relax, unwind, be at one with nature and savour its beauty. First you have to remove the weeds that are clogging up the ground and choking it. They are blocking all the beautiful flowers from growing and smothering the flowers that have managed to bloom.

Your irrational beliefs are the weeds, the ones that are prohibiting your garden from being at its best. Your rational beliefs are the flowers, the ones that help you to enhance your garden. Examine every belief so you can determine if they are weeds or flowers. If they are weeds pull them out and throw them away. Allow the flowers to bloom to their full potential and plant new ones, so that you can create a beautiful, healthy, joyful garden.

TASK FOUR: *WHAT ARE MY BELIEFS?*

Using your diary make a list of all the beliefs you can think of in relation to

   A) Food
   B) Your Weight
   C) Eating

As an example - Food:
     I believe food is there to comfort me when I am upset
     I believe food will solve all my problems – etc etc

Make a list of 10 or 15 beliefs in each category or as many as you can come up with.

When you have finished this list look at each belief individually and identify which ones have contributed to you being fat. Mark each one with an X. These are the beliefs that have brought you to a place where you are not happy. They are predominantly the reasons why you have those feelings that you identified in task 1.

Now look at the list again and mark with a tick any beliefs that will help to enhance your life and support your new goal? Which of these beliefs, are based on reality? Will they promote new healthy feelings and behaviours?

Take the beliefs that you marked with a tick, write them onto a new page entitled, My New Life Enhancing Beliefs.

Now go back to those you marked with an X. These are the ones that need to be "reframed"; these beliefs need to be completely transformed so that they can become new Life Enhancing Beliefs.

These beliefs are based on your experience of a situation. However, the facts of the situation are lost because of the interpretation you gave it at the time. This then became your belief. For example, every time you were upset as a child your mother gave you chocolate. Your interpretation of this situation could lead you to believe that "Chocolate takes the pain away; it makes me feel better when I am sad".

The fact is, chocolate served as a temporary distraction from the pain, causing you to believe the chocolate made you feel better. I have worked with many people who would have a belief very similar to this one. However, when I ask any of them the question, "Does chocolate really take away the pain that you are feeling?", every one of them says - no! So how rational is this belief? It is completely irrational. Chocolate or food does not take away stress, sadness, loneliness, or any other emotion. It serves as a temporary distraction from it. The emotions are still there after the food is eaten and very often the feeling of guilt is there too.

So in this case how would you reframe this belief? To reframe a belief you have first of all to be sure of the new one. You have to be sure it is based on fact and is reliable.

It helps to ask yourself a number of questions in order to challenge the belief.

Example,

- ❖ When I feel sad and eat 4 bars of chocolate do I actually stop feeling sad?

- ❖ How do I actually feel after eating the chocolate?

- ❖ Could doing something else make me feel better?

- ❖ What could I do other than eat chocolate?

When you have challenged your belief and discover that it doesn't serve you and help you, it is time to change it – move on to one that does. So in this case, for example, you might change your belief to:

"Eating is an ineffective way to deal with emotional pain or discomfort".

Now you have identified the limiting belief, you can see that it is not serving you effectively - and you have challenged it! You have reframed it in a way that will serve you and help you to achieve your new goal and new life.

Now do this with your X marked beliefs: and turn them into your new life enhancing beliefs.

STRATEGY FOUR

Your old beliefs have been part of your world for a long time, either consciously or unconsciously. They will not just disappear because you have new ones. You will need to keep your new beliefs in your consciousness and be aware of them at all times and use them. When you stop using the old ones and keep practicing the new ones then they will become automatic in time.

TASK FOUR part 2: *MY NEGATIVE SELF TALK*

For that negative self talk, have your diary close at hand and when you hear that voice trying to restrict you and sabotage your efforts, identify what is being said.

Write it down.

Challenge it.

Write down your challenging questions and your answers.

Ask the right questions; find the right answers; defeat the negative talk.

STRATEGY FOUR part 2

Remember: anything going on in your head that is not contributing to your happiness and fulfilment is only going to make you unhappy and unfulfilled.

You have set your goal now, you know how fed up you are being fat and you don't want to stay like this. You know what you want to achieve. Any thoughts and beliefs that you have that don't support you to do this are useless. They are no longer required. No matter what the beliefs and thoughts are, if they don't serve to enhance your life, you know what to do: bin them!

Feelings are Feelings are Feelings:

---

*"There is a great deal of pain in life
and perhaps the only pain
that can be avoided is the
pain of trying to avoid pain"*

R.D Laing

Feelings are just that, feelings. They are physical sensations that are not connected with sight, hearing, taste or smell. While our external senses are needed as guides to our external world and they steer us away from physical harm, our feelings act as our guide to our internal world and are also attempting to steer us away from harm.

However, while many of us would automatically trust our senses to lead us away from danger, e.g. a fire; we can see it, hear it, and smell it: but when it comes to feelings we often try and bury them with food. We are too afraid to face the feeling and feel it. It might be too painful so we avoid it, but as RD Laing, a British psychoanalyst has said, the pain of trying to avoid pain is actually the only pain we can avoid. We can't avoid pain in life; it is a natural part of life. We can, however choose how much we let it affect our lives. You can chose to let sadness turn to depression or anger to rage - uncertainty to hopelessness, fear into terror, or envy into hatred.

Allow your feelings to be! Acknowledge them; accept them; and feel them. They are there for a reason; they are telling you what is going on in your internal world. It is just as important to feel sadness as it is happiness. Yet we generally don't stop ourselves from feeling the good feelings in the way we do with the bad. Why?

There are 2 reasons:
1) As Freud identified in his Pleasure Principle, we strive to move towards pleasure and away from pain.

2) Because we have a belief that inhibits us from feeling them. Again we are back to the irrational beliefs.

 In relation to our feelings we may believe for whatever reason that,

- It is weak to cry
- I should always be in good form
- Emotional pain serves no function
- Strong people don't show their emotions
- I have to stay strong for everyone else
- I couldn't bear painful emotions

These beliefs are a result of your interpretation of an event or situation in the past. They possibly served you in some way at the time but now these beliefs are only going to hold you back from being truly happy. Emotional wellbeing is a result of acknowledging and experiencing your feelings. They are your very own guide to your internal world and if you listen to them you will develop a great relationship with your own body.

Feelings are your messages about how something has impacted on you. By allowing yourself to feel, you are allowing the emotion to run its course and dissipate. Burying or hiding your feelings will only result in storing them for another day, when they can possibly erupt even stronger and more painfully. I know this from personal experience. Having had 4 miscarriages over 15 months I became very well acquainted with many painful emotions: sadness, grief, disappointment, anger, distress; to name just a few. Sometimes I was hit with one at a time, other occasions by many together.

Each miscarriage was as dreadful as the last. Once I discovered with each new pregnancy that the development of the baby had stopped I knew I was faced with going into that terrible distress once more.

I had the choice to do something to take all the elements of the pain away, to hide it or bury it; anything to avoid that much heartache again or I could face it head on and deal with it. I chose to deal with it. Although the pain didn't get any easier, each time I felt a little bit stronger, knowing that I had the inner resources to get through it.

Burying the pain or fighting it would not have made me stronger. Something devastating had happened to me 4 times. My body was responding. To get to a better place I knew I had to go through it. I had to feel the pain. So I did. I cried when I felt like crying, which was most of the time for a while. I allowed the anger to come out when I could feel it inside, I let the disappointment out and I let myself grieve.

Once the emotions were given release, they eased with time. Every day became easier, every day I felt a little bit stronger. Once the emotions had eased significantly I was then in a place where I could put myself back together and focus on what brought me joy and happiness. The pain had served its purpose. I had to grieve and say goodbye to my 4 babies before I could move forward in a healthy way. I focused on my healthy happy 2 year old, my loving husband, our wonderful friends and the active fulfilling life I have.

I know now that if I am to face a painful time again in the future that I have the strength to get through it. I can look to my past and see that I got through pain and that I can do it again if I need to. I know I have the essential tools. By knowing this I can look to the future with optimism and hope, without letting the fear of possible pain stop me from living my life as fully as I possibly can. I make plans and set myself new goals all the time so that I have a wonderful and compelling future. There are always options and choices. We don't have to stay in a painful place and suffer. There are always choices we can make to take ourselves to a happier place.

It's amazing how a painful experience can cause you to look at life in a very different way. I am now more appreciative of all the wonderful things in my life; that I am in fact so lucky to have what I have. I know how important the little tiny precious moments are, that I have with my family and friends; or those wonderful times when I am surrounded by the wonders of Mother Nature's creations. All are things that can be bypassed in the hectic way of life our society demands.

Emotions can act as a wake-up call in life, they shout at you to tell you to stop and take heed. If you are stressed your body will tell you, but will you take the time to listen? Take the time to slow down and feel the stress so that you can identify it? Find out where the source lies? When you know the cause you can work on it, to reduce the stress that will invariably take its toll on you physically and psychologically.

While food might serve as a temporary distraction from painful emotions, it doesn't eradicate them. They will still be there when you stop eating. The relief is short lived, the emotion is still there and your waistline is getting fatter. And then there are the emotions that come with eating to avoid or bury emotions - the guilt, the shame, the hopelessness; they emerge to compound the situation even further, making the situation so difficult that it seems there is no way out of the vicious circle.

There *is* a way out. Manage your emotions. Acknowledge that you are feeling something, identify what emotion it is, feel it, allow it to be and come out the other side. Also looking at where the emotion is coming from is very useful. Is it connected to your belief system, your behaviour?

One of my clients felt down and depressed a lot. When he felt this way he ate. He ate anything, anything that was in the house. If there was nothing there he would drive to the petrol station at any time of the night and buy, sometimes, a couple of bags of food. He would eat until he could not eat anymore. He said it made him feel better. There was a certainty and a comfort with food.

He knew he would get a distraction from his emotions. Albeit temporary it was still a distraction. It was also company. However, at the end of the binge he still felt depressed, but now even worse because he knew the eating was not the answer. He felt full but empty at the same time. All it was doing was making him fatter.

I asked him what the cause of the initial depression was. What was the trigger? What happened in his day to cause him to feel this way? He wasn't sure of the answers, so I asked him to keep a journal for the week, to take note of what happened. In the next session he said he felt the trigger came when he thought about how alone he was in his life that he became depressed. More often than not, it would be triggered by his colleagues talking about going out socialising at night or at the weekends with their partners or friends. It reminded him that he had no partner and virtually no friends. He was lonely.

However, despite this realisation he felt unable to do anything about it. He didn't go out. He believed he was not interesting enough to be around other people. What could he talk about? It basically came down to his self esteem, his beliefs about himself. He believed he had nothing to offer. Through coaching he worked on challenging this belief. He binned it and made new rational beliefs for himself. His weight was part of this also and by losing some weight and working on his beliefs, he would not now think of sitting at home on a Saturday night with bags of food from the local petrol station. He is too busy living in the company of his friends.

My client's life was a vicious cycle. He felt depressed so ate to relieve it, but in turn his excessive eating was making him more depressed. He could not see a way out of this cycle even though it was making him miserable. When he was able to figure out what was causing the initial trigger to this cycle he was then able to break it down and uncover the irrational beliefs that he had and subsequently work on challenging and replacing them .This lead him to a happier place; a place where he didn't need food to make him feel better.

An important thing to highlight here is that my client was getting something from his behaviour. He was in fact gaining in a way from his eating. The majority of the time we are gaining something from our habits, they are protecting us in some way or they are meeting our needs in some way. Not necessarily in a positive way, but meeting them all the same.

There are important questions to ask yourself:

- "What is my reward for behaving in this way?"

- "What am I getting from behaving this way?"

- "What needs am I satisfying?"

The answers to these questions are vital because if you are gaining in some way from your behaviours, parting with them will be difficult until you find an alternative. You need to replace it with something that will give you what you need. Otherwise you face an inevitable internal conflict. The desire to change and achieve your goal will be sabotaged by your stronger desire to keep getting whatever it is you derive from your current behaviours. It will prevent you from making real changes.

The Six Basic Human Needs

Anthony Robbins, the American peak performance coach, has influenced the lives of millions of people, throughout the world and has combined his expertise with Dr. Cloe Madanes, a world renowned innovator and teacher of family and brief therapy. Together they created the Robbins-Madanes Centre for Strategic Intervention, which extracts the most practical and effective forms of strategic action from disciplines, such as, Ericksonian therapy, strategic family therapy, human needs psychology, organisational psychology and many more. The Robbins-Madanes tradition of Strategic Intervention is called Human Needs Psychology.

Within this they believe that we all possess Six Basic Human needs, which are the driving force in our lives. As human beings we are striving to meet all six needs but there are two that we usually value more than the others.

Knowing which needs are driving you the most can help you understand why you make the choices you do and gain some insight into your emotional patterns. Our actions, behaviours and beliefs are what we choose so that we can meet the needs most important to us. These are what Human Needs Psychology defines as the vehicles we use to meet our needs. These vehicles can be positive or negative, they can either support you in achieving your goals or they can be destructive in the long term: in other words, they can make you Fat and Fed Up!

Have a look at the six needs and ask yourself what part they play in your life:

1. <u>Certainty/Comfort</u> - Do you like stability in your life? Do you like to know that your basic necessities in life are certain, e.g. food, home, possessions. Do you enjoy having control over your world?
2. <u>Uncertainty/Variety</u> – Do you like to change your state, to exercise your emotions and your body? Do you like variety and seek it through means such as a change of scene, physical activity, mood swings, entertainment, extreme sports, food?
3. <u>Significance</u> – Do you like to feel important, unique, special or needed? Do you enjoy recognition from others?
4. <u>Connection/Love</u> – Do you like to feel connected with someone or something, e.g. a person, an ideal, a value or a habit?
5. <u>Growth</u> – Everything in the universe is either growing or dying. Do you enjoy expanding your capacities, skills, interests?
6. <u>Contribution</u> – Do you enjoy contributing to others? Do you want to contribute something of value to help others?

The client I described above was eating excessively to cover up and hide his emotions; he was able to avoid them by eating. He also said he felt safe when he was eating; a certainty and security came with it. He knew what he was going to get.

It was also the path of least resistance for him; he didn't have to face reality when he was hiding behind food.

There are many needs that you may have that your behaviour is meeting.

- Maybe you feel protected by the layer of fat that you carry around and feel certain and safe with it?

- Maybe the attention that it brings in the form of concern from others makes you feel significant and you like this?

Whatever needs you are satisfying you need to recognise it because your behaviour is taking you to a place that you are not happy. The price that you are paying for satisfying your needs is too great. Once you identify what needs you are trying to satisfy you will be able to look for new healthy ways of meeting them that don't bring such negative consequences.

"Happy is the man
who has been able to learn
the causes of things"

Virgil

Take the time for the next task to help you to discover what it is that is that triggers the emotions that lead you to eating. Also give yourself the time to work out what needs you are meeting by your actions and your behaviours. This new awareness about your eating will help you to make the changes that support your new goal.

TASK FOUR part 3: *MY TRIGGERS AND NEEDS*

Take time to discover your triggers. Use your journal and write down what happens when you feel like eating in response to your emotions.

What emotions are stirring inside you?
Connect with them. Identify them. Feel them.

What caused these emotions to stir up inside you?
>   Was it a specific incident?
>   Was it a person?
>   Was it a series of incidents?

What was your reaction?
>   What were you thinking in response to this trigger?
>   What beliefs can you identify in connection to this reaction?

Are these beliefs rational?
Are they irrational?

Have you the power to change something about this incident to make sure a similar incident does not reoccur?
Will you need to change how you think about it, i.e., your beliefs?

My Needs: (Use the 6 Basic Needs to guide you)
What needs are you satisfying by your behaviour?
Does your behaviour make you feel Safe? Secure? Protected? Significant?

Ask yourself why it is important to feel Safe? Significant? Protected? etc
What else can you do to meet these needs besides eating?
Make a list of your options.

STRATEGY FOUR part 3

No matter what happens to you in life that is difficult and causes you to feel pain, stress, anger, etc, repeat this process to help you to deal with it.

Identify what happened to cause the emotion.
Identify what belief you had around it.
Check if this belief is useful to you or hindering you.

Is the situation something that can be changed or is it something that requires you to change the way you think about it.
Either way, by building an awareness of how things, people, situations and events impact on you in an emotional way, you will develop the power to deal with them in a healthy, progressive, empowering way.

I C A N C o a c h i n g P u b l i s h i n g

Feel your feelings and allow them to be. Ignoring them or burying them under a pile of food is not going to be conducive to a happy life. You now have the tools you need to overcome the old reactions you have had to feeling difficult emotions.

So far you have identified how you feel being fat. You decided on what you want to achieve from this process, your goal. You identified your habits and patterns that have lead to your body shape. Now you also have an understanding of the importance and the impact of your belief system on your emotions and your behaviours.

Use this new understanding to work on the habits and patterns that you identified in task three. The next task helps you to put everything you have worked on in the previous tasks together to give you a greater understanding of your world.

TASK FOUR part 4: *THE CAUSES OF MY BEHAVIOUR*

Revisit the list of habits, patterns and behaviours you made earlier in your journal.

Look at each one. Decide if they are habits, i.e., an automatic response to a situation from years of conditioning, e.g. not eating breakfast, for no reason other than you never do. Or decide if they are behaviours in response to an irrational belief that you have.

Then bearing in mind the beliefs and triggers you have discovered in this section, try and match them up to each of your behaviours. Be mindful also of the needs you want to satisfy, that you have identified.

Example –
> You overeat when you have had a difficult day; (your *behaviour*)
> You have the *belief* that food is a way to relieve stress.
> Stress is your *trigger* to eat binge eating.
> Food is meeting your *need* for comfort and safety from the difficult day.

You might have reframed your belief to *"Food does not relieve stress; there are many other ways that I can choose to relax and de-stress"*. Then make a list of other ways to relieve stress.

Do this exercise with all of the habits and behaviours you identified. Attach all of your new life enhancing beliefs to your existing behaviours and find alternatives to the habits that you possess.

STRATEGY FOUR part 4

When you find yourself tempted to behave in an old way,
repeat the new belief that you have formed.

Do this as many times as it takes for you to act in the new
way, which is going to help you to achieve your goals.

There has been quite a lot in this section for you to take in, understand and work on.

✓ I believe however, it is the most important section of this book;

Without the understanding and insight you have gained here, any attempts to lose weight would be doomed, like they have been in the past. When you understand why you do things, then you can change what is making you unhappy. If you don't give yourself the time to discover the cause of something, then how can you truly understand it, and change it for the better?

To recap your progress to date: in **Step 1**, you began by identifying how being fat makes you feel. You know what you want to leave behind and never have to face again. In **Step 2**, you set your goal, you decided what exactly it is you want to achieve and when you want to achieve it by.
In **Step 3**, you identified what behaviours, habits and patterns have led you to put on weight. You have learned what worked for you in the past and what didn't work for you as ways of losing weight and why.

In **Step 4**, you have worked intensively on your mind in relation to eating, food and your weight. You identified your irrational beliefs and worked on changing them to new life enhancing beliefs that are going to help you to

---

achieve your goals as opposed to stopping you. You know what negative self talk is and how you can challenge it and change it. You know what beliefs are responsible for your behaviour and you have identified the habits that are contributing to your weight gain. You possess new beliefs that make this behaviour and these habits redundant and instead promote healthy feelings and behaviours.

You know what needs you are trying to satisfy by your behaviour and you now have other options available to you to meet these needs in a healthier way.

The work you have done in this section has been based around what you have been doing to date to feed your mind. Eating in response to your head only makes you fat, but you now hold the tools that you need to avoid this happening again in the future.

Now it is time to learn how to *Eat Right*.

Chapter 11:

Step 5: Eat Right:

Eating right requires knowing what a balanced healthy diet is. We all know, despite what we think, what are the right things to be eating:

-   Which is a healthier snack, an apple or a bar of chocolate?

-   Which is a healthier drink, a bottle of water or a can of fizzy drink?

-   Which is a healthier dinner, a homemade meal or a ready-made processed microwavable meal?

I don't need to tell you. We all know the healthier options but do we always choose them?

No we don't! But you know what, it is ok to choose some chocolate or a piece of cake or whatever you fancy: every now and again. This process is not about denial. It is about consciousness and awareness. Everything you do from now on is going to be the result of a conscious decision, a considered choice - not as a response to a bad habit.

The purpose of this step, *Eat Right*, is to help you to create your own new norm of eating: a healthy, nutritious, balanced, tasty way of eating. This norm that you will create for yourself will be the basis for your daily food intake. You can choose what food you want to include and yes, even some "nice" things.

Possibly at this stage you might be thinking, "<u>Some</u> nice things! If I was allowed to eat nice things then I would never stop". Or maybe you are thinking, "I know what food I should be eating I just don't know how much, my portions are always too big!"

If your negative self-talk (aka your gremlin or your monster), is raising his head when we are addressing food and telling you things like, " you have no control over nice food", then you must use what you learned in *Think Right*, to identify the irrational beliefs and challenge the self defeating talk. Listen to whatever is emerging in your head. Identify it, feel the emotions that are rising up - break it down and get to the roots. You have the tools now to sabotage the saboteur. Keep using them every time you hear the negative talk or feel like doing something that does not support your goal or promote healthy emotions or behaviour.

You are now going to decide what you are going to eat and as you learn how much to eat, without counting calories or points. Your days of counting and denial are gone; it's time for learning something new that is going to help you to achieve your goal.

To do this you will:

a) Re-educate yourself as to what a healthy diet is,
b) Become a conscious eater.
c) Connect with your body.

What does a healthy diet include?

I am not a nutritionist or qualified to advise people on what they should eat. Anyway if I was to write 5 or 10 pages of lists of do's and don'ts about what foods to eat, I would just become like all the other weight loss books and diets you have spent money on. This way of losing weight is different.

You have not spent the money on this book and spent the time to read it to be told by another person what you *should* and *should not* be eating. You have tried this before and it didn't work. Instead you are learning how to develop your own way of eating healthily every day.

The power of coaching lies in its ability to help people to help themselves, to empower people to find their own answers to their questions. One very powerful question worth asking yourself now is,

"What can I eat now that is consistent with who I am now and what I want in my life?"

You are creating a new you by creating new beliefs and you have a specific goal you want to achieve. Bear this in mind when you are creating your new eating plan.

What I will recommend, and it is what I use when coaching my clients, is the food pyramid. The food pyramid is an illustration of what a balanced healthy diet looks like and it is designed to make healthy eating easier. It is recommended by the World Health Organisation. It is a brilliant tool for sensible sustainable eating.

In summary, it is a pyramid divided into 5 shelves. Each shelf holds the recommended amount of food from the main food groups we can eat as part of a healthy eating plan.

1) The bottom shelf contains carbohydrates, such as bread, pasta, cereal, potatoes etc. We are encouraged to eat 6+ servings a day.
2) Fruits and vegetables make up the next shelf. It is recommended we eat 5+ servings of these daily.
3) Dairy is on the next shelf, 2-3 servings are important daily.
4) Meat is the next group of which we are encouraged to eat 2-3 servings for protein and iron.

5) The top of the pyramid contains oils, sweets, chocolate, and saturated fats. It is recommended that we only include small amounts of these in our diets.

It also recommends drinking at least 8 cups of water a day.

(To obtain a full illustrated copy of the food pyramid, just Google, The Food Pyramid. There are numerous places from which you can download your own full colour copy.)

What I love about the food pyramid way of eating is that it encourages us to have a little of everything. So you achieve a balanced healthy diet, even including a little of what you fancy.

The food pyramid will help you to create your own way of healthy eating. The guidelines are there as to the right foods, you can mix match as it suits you.

> If you have a specific food allergy or intolerance, I recommend you speak to your doctor or a qualified professional knowledgeable in the area to help you to put your eating plan together.

I highly recommend using the food pyramid as your guideline for your new healthy eating plan. If you combine all the recommendations in a way that you enjoy, then you will have created a hugely valuable tool. This tool will help you to achieve your goals and also help you maintain it for life - so that "dieting" and losing weight will never have to be part of your life again.

Using what you learned in Step 2 about your eating choices for losing weight, use the positives and the negatives you learned to help you in choosing your new eating plan. For example, you might have used a diet that required counting calories or points, you might have liked the recipes they offered but couldn't stick to the counting regime. Whatever eating guidelines you use make sure they do not incorporate things from the past that did not work for you.

Don't allow restrictions and denial to become part of your plan, otherwise you are on a "diet" and we know those don't work in the long run.

This step is about creating a new healthy lifestyle change, bringing new positive tasty options into your daily eating plan. Create a plan that includes a little of everything.

Many of my clients find the best tool they use in relation to eating right is planning. They plan their meals each week, taking one week at a time. They plan what each dinner is going to be at the beginning of the week and buy accordingly.

They check what is coming up for them during the week in terms of commitments that might cause them to deviate from their regular eating pattern and they plan a response to this:

- ✓ Therefore, if they know they are going to be late at work they might cook their meal the night before so they merely have to heat it up once they get home.
- ✓ Or they might take healthy snacks to work to keep them going until they get home and to eliminate the temptation of the vending machine at work.

Not forgetting that this is in essence a "how to lose weight" book, we can't ignore that to lose weight, you need to be using more calories than you are consuming. This however does not mean that you have to be counting the calories you are eating and monitoring the ones you are burning. That's what you did before and it didn't work. Eliminating the bad habits and patterns in your life that are somewhat responsible for the weight gain in the first place, will help you to lose weight immediately. Combining this with eating healthy food in the quantities that your body needs and moving right (which you will work on in step 6) you will lose weight and achieve the body shape that you want.

So before we move onto learning how much to eat, complete task five to formulate your new eating plan. Maybe you feel that you already eat well, that your main meals are not the reason for your weight gain, this maybe so but I would encourage you to complete this exercise even if just as a review of your eating. Maybe you might find ways to improve it a little bit.

TASK FIVE: *MY NEW EATING PLAN*

Plan what you are going to eat for each meal for 7 days. Use the food pyramid (or any alternative healthy eating guidelines you have researched), together with what you have learned from the past, about what works and what doesn't work for you.

Day 1: Breakfast: _____
      Lunch: _____
      Dinner: _____

Day 2: Breakfast: _____
      Lunch: _____
      Dinner: _____

And so on, for 7 days

Even if you have not eaten 3 meals a day up to now – if you have skipped breakfast or never eaten a dinner - include them in the plan. If skipping a meal has been a habit for you, you possibly have identified it as one of your habits or patterns when doing task three: and you may have worked out

---

I C A N C o a c h i n g P u b l i s h i n g

why you do it. If not, now would be a good time to use the tool and work backwards to find out why you are doing this. When you know why, you are in a better position to change it.

Make your eating plan for one week at a time. You might find at the end of the week there are things you would like to vary and change, to make it better. Keep making these plans for a few weeks until your new way of eating have become automatic.

When you are familiar with the types of food that you have chosen, you can decide easily what you will have for your meals on a daily bases including these foods.

STRATEGY FIVE

If you have a bad day or weekend or go overboard on a holiday, don't let this throw you back into old habits. Your new eating plan is your new habit, go back to this.

Make it your "norm" that you will return to.

The healthy choices will, in a short time, undo the temporary bad ones you make, returning to bad choices full time will inevitably make you fatter!

Now you know what you are going to eat every day, the next step is to learn how to eat properly. This might sound a bit basic but it is something that many of us have forgotten to do in our adulthood. As babies we knew when we were hungry, we would cry and we would be fed. We would stop when our bellies were full and we were satisfied until we felt hunger again, when we would proceed once again to make it known to our parents we needed to be fed.

As children we listened to our bodies. We looked for food when we were hungry, we stopped when we are no longer hungry, and direct our attention to something else - playing with toys, playing with friends - and continued to do so until our tummies once more tell us it is time for fuel. Those of us that have become fat somewhere along the line stopped eating just to fuel our bodies and started eating for other reasons, like the ones you have identified in step 4. You know what your reasons are: this is what you are identifying and challenging. Now it is time to learn to reconnect with your body and feed it for the right reasons.

Eat Right! Feed your Stomach not your Mind!

Outside of eating the wrong foods another contributing factor to being fat is eating to satisfy our minds not our stomachs. You have identified what your reasons for eating are. Some that my clients have identified include:

- "I feel like something nice to eat"
- "I have had a bad day I deserve something nice"
- "It is one o clock, I should be having lunch"
- "I am at a buffet, I am supposed to eat loads"
- "I will eat more now so I won't be hungry later"
- "I am out for a nice meal, I am going to have all 3 courses and eat it all, I am paying for it after all"

These are just an example of ways we feed our mind; there is no connection with our stomachs here. When we are not listening to our bodies telling us when to eat, we are far more at risk of eating too much and of eating the wrong foods.

To avoid this happening we must learn how to listen to our body and more importantly trust our bodies to know what it needs. The best way to do this is to start with listening to the physical signs of hunger. Get connected to your body, hear the sounds of hunger, feel the signals of its need for food. A great tool to help you to do this is to use the Hunger Scale, see page 107. Identify what happens to your body when you start to feel hungry, when you are starving, when you are satisfied and when you are full.

When you are able to identify the stages of the scale within your body, you will be far less inclined to leave it too late to eat, which will only lead to eating the wrong foods for a quick fix. It will also help you to stop eating as soon as you feel satisfied, which in turn will stop you from overeating.

- ✓ It really is that straight forward, eat when you are hungry, and stop when you are satisfied.

Your task for this section is to use the hunger scale below, on page 107, each time you eat, for as long as it takes to become automatic. Copy it if it helps and keep it in your wallet or purse or on the fridge door, somewhere that you can refer to it quickly and easily when you need it.

The challenge here is going to be, finding the trust that you have lost in your body. If you have been eating to feed your mind for years then you have stopped listening to your stomach. Food is for fuelling and nourishing your body, nothing else. You give it what it needs when it needs it.
- ✓ How do you know what it needs and when it needs it?
- ✓ You listen to it.

How do you know when you are tired? How do you know when you are feeling sick? How do you know when you need to use the toilet? You know these things because you listen to what your body is telling you. It gives you signals; you listen, hear and respond in the appropriate way depending on the situation. If you ignored these signals there would be serious health repercussions.

So why do we fail to listen to our body when it comes to eating? Well mainly for the reasons we have already described. We have the ability when we are young but somewhere along the line we start eating for reasons other than fuel and nutrition. At this stage you will have identified what your reasons are.

When we put on weight we look for ways to lose it, reaching for the automatic solution of the diet. What the diet tells is not to listen to our bodies. The diet tells us when to eat, what to eat and how much to eat. We are told to eat the "good" food and stay away from the "bad" food. We choose weight loss products that promise to make us lose 10lbs in 10 days. We opt for shakes instead of real food.

Then when the diet comes to an end we still don't know how to eat properly so we go back to what we did before: because that is all we know and we carry on putting weight back on, while beating ourselves up for yet another diet failure.

Ask yourself this,

How can anything that goes against all that is natural work in the long term?

The answer is, it can't! Therefore, you were doomed for failure before you even started your diets.

Now use the hunger scale to reconnect with your body. Your body will tell you when it is hungry, when it has had enough and when it is thirsty. You merely have to listen and recognise the signals. Hear what they are telling you and give your body what it needs.

TASK FIVE part 2: *APPLYING THE HUNGER SCALE*

Use the hunger scale every day for the next 2 weeks. Every time you eat identify what number you are at.

Did you wait too long to eat and eat at 1 or 2?

Did you ignore your body and eat until you were so full you were at a 9 or a 10?

This will take a lot of practice if you are not used to eating this way. You have been eating a specific way for a while now, so it will take time to change it, but at this stage you have many tools to help you and it will become natural in time.

You have formulated your own eating plan and you have identified your eating habits. Your new eating plan has been based on three meals a day: no more skipping breakfast or eating too much at dinner. Now it is time to use the hunger scale to decide if this is what is going to suit you or if you need to make some adjustments.

- Use your new eating plan for a week at a time. Use the hunger scale in conjunction with it each day. Eat the meals you have planned.

If you are someone that has never eaten breakfast and does not feel hungry in the morning, this is because you have trained your metabolism not to wake up when you do. It is another habit you have taught your body.

Many of us that are trying to lose weight feel that skipping breakfast is one less meal so less calories. It is less calories in the day per se: but it tells your metabolism to slow down and thus burn less calories. That is defeating the purpose of helping you to lose weight. Inevitably, you will be starving by lunch time and more than likely eat too much and of the wrong food. It doesn't work and it's not healthy or natural.

Even if you feel you couldn't eat a breakfast this is the one time I will say "go against what your body is telling you, just in the short term". Even by eating a small piece of fruit or a yogurt, something light, then your body will start responding and getting used to food in the morning. You will kick start your metabolism which will in turn work for you throughout the day, burning more calories for energy and also giving your brain the fuel and energy it needs to tackle the day ahead.

Stop eating when you are satisfied, when you no longer feel hungry. In between meals listen to your body. Ask yourself - am I feeling hungry between meals? Am I hungry after my dinner? Am I too hungry to last from lunch time to dinner time? Am I just starting to get hungry when I get home in time for dinner? Am I perfectly satisfied between each meal? Am I hungry or thirsty?

You will see how 3 meals works for you or if some days you need an extra snack to keep going. The important thing is to let your body decide what it needs. When you have identified what and how much food your body needs, then plan around it. When you are shopping include what snacks you like and will need for the week.

Do you like fruit/dried fruit/yogurts? What is your body looking for?

Now you know what to eat; how much of it to eat; and when to eat it.

Eat Consciously

Before we leave *Eat Right* it is important to look at what it means to eat consciously. So far you have made the conscious decision to make a change. You are not happy as you are now and you know something has to change or it is going to get worse. You have set your goal. You are now very clear about what you want to achieve and you know how much it will mean to you.

You have identified what beliefs, habits and patterns have contributed to you having the body you have now. You have learned how to change these beliefs and how to deal with your emotions. You have made your new eating plan and you now know how to connect with your body to eat the right amounts at the right times. It is now important to keep all of this in your consciousness, in your awareness so that your new changes will be easier to make. The success of the new changes you have chosen to make is dependent on the decisions you make every day. In an ideal world all of the choices you made as a result of this book will go perfectly to plan; nothing will happen to divert you from your new course. This is not a perfect world! Things can, and do, happen every day that challenge us or upset us or cause us to question our choices.

No matter what you are faced with from now on that might impact on the success of your goal, there is no need for regret or guilt so long as you make a conscious decision for every action that you take.

For example, at this stage of their coaching many of my clients panic a little bit about events or situations that are to come in their lives. They are still at the early stage of their changes and their new habits have not yet become automatic. They become fearful that an event like a wedding or a holiday or a weekend away is going to push them back into their old habits and everything will have been a waste.

All you can do is make conscious decisions in the situation you are in. After all this is about changing your lifestyle not about being on a diet. You are working towards making a new "norm" for yourself. No matter what situation you are faced with remember life is full of these situations and life is to be enjoyed.

Whether you are on your holidays or at a wedding when it comes to eating and drinking make a conscious decision at the time, ask yourself, "Right now, at this moment, do I want the glass of beer or the bowl of ice-cream?"

If the answer is "yes I really do want this", then you have checked with yourself first and in that moment you want some ice-cream. You have not taken it just because you are where you are, or because you always do when you are on holidays.

In the past in these situations did you ever find yourself saying, "I am on holidays, I will start my diet when I go home" or "I will eat what I want during my weekend away and I will be good from Monday.".........

.... This is diet mentality; that you start and stop doing something. Your new mentality is based around a new way of life, that will be permanent. If you find it difficult in any of these situations, break it down. Only think about the very moment you are in, the decision you are faced with. Don't think about later in the day, tomorrow or next Monday: the only moment that matters is now. Think about your goal and what you want. Make a conscious decision about what you do or don't do. Don't do something because you have always done it, those days are behind you.

You have now chosen to be in control of everything you think, feel and do.

When you are aware of what you are doing then you will be less inclined to overdo it. Even if you do feel like you overdid it, despite making a conscious decision, treat it as part of the situation that it is. Weddings and holidays do not happen every day. They are a natural part of life and there to be enjoyed. The important thing is not to let these indulgences distract you from your new healthy way of life, which you have chosen. As you have learned from Strategy Five all the "rights" that you do will in a very short time undo any "wrongs" that you make along the way.

Also, eating consciously involves connecting with food that is in your mouth. While food is for fuel it can still be enjoyed. Experience each mouthful that you take. Savour it! Enjoy it! Many of my clients say to me, "Catherine, I just love food, I eat because I love it." This is perfectly fine, in fact it is great. Again eating is a part of life, it is how we socialise, how we celebrate, part of how we can experience different cultures. I said earlier food is for fuel and nourishment and nothing else. This however does not mean that we cannot enjoy this fuel. In fact it is important that we do. However, it is not a licence to eat fast food everyday because you love it. In fact even if you did this every day for a week, I can guarantee that your body would start telling you that it wanted something different. And if you listened to your body you would stop doing it even if you loved the food. You can enjoy a perfectly healthy way of eating that supports your goal of your ideal body shape and still enjoy your food.

Of all the great healthy foods that are out there, choose the food that you like. You now know what a balanced diet looks like; you have seen the food pyramid. However, you always have choices. You might not like potatoes, this is fine; there are options; pasta, rice etc. You might not like milk, but you can eat cheese and yogurts. Whatever it is choose the foods you like and when you are eating it enjoy it. Savour the flavours, the taste and the texture. If you are not enjoying it there is nothing wrong with leaving it and choosing something else.

Eating for the sake of it will not bring you satisfaction. It is important to feel satisfied by your meals both physically and experientially. If you eat a meal that you didn't like or enjoy chances are you will want to go looking for something else that you can enjoy even if you are not hungry.

A way to ensure that you are gaining in every way from what you are eating is to eat consciously. Don't sit in front of the television when you are eating, be aware of what you are eating and enjoy it, experience it and savour it. Granted it might not always be possible to eat slowly and consciously, e.g., if you're eating at your desk, when you are hurrying out in the morning - but always choose the food you prefer and when you can, enjoy it for what it is.

Allow it to satisfy you on every level.

Eat with awareness; make your decisions with awareness, not out of habit. Connect with and listen to your body, don't beat yourself up for enjoying your life, enjoy the events and occasions in your life for what they are. Have a healthy natural way of eating and living and you will never be fat and have to worry about your weight again.

The Hunger Scale – Connecting with your Body

1 ------ Sick → You are so hungry you feel sick & could eat anything

2------ Irritable → You need to eat and quickly

3------ Hungry → Your tummy is rumbling

4------ Pangs → You are slightly hungry and starting to feel like food

5------ Satisfied → You are just right, comfortable and content

6------ Full → You can feel the food against your stomach

7------ Too full → You can feel the food pushing your stomach

8------ Bloated → You can feel your stomach stretched

9------ Uncomfortable → Your stomach hurts and your clothes feel tight

10------ Sick → You actually feel sick from too much food

KEY:

1 & 2 - Avoid waiting until you are starving to eat – you are more likely to eat food that gives you a short term sugar fix for energy.

3 –Now is a good time to eat

4- Your body is telling you it is going to need food soon, time to start thinking about getting some good food

5- Now is time to stop eating. You cannot feel your stomach anymore. You are neither hungry nor full.

6, 7, 8 & 9 – these are all the signals of overeating. Once you can feel your stomach, i.e. the food pressing against it, then you have exceeded your stomachs capacity. Your body doesn't need that much food and it certainly doesn't need to feel so stuffed with food that you feel sick.

Learn to listen to your body. Practice eating when you are hungry and stop when you are satisfied. With practice it will become a natural way of being, of living. This technique will be responsible for maintaining your desired body shape.

Now that you have your new eating plan in place and you know how to eat properly and consciously, let's move onto Step 6, *Move Right.*

Chapter 12:

Step 6: Move Right!

To lose weight it is necessary to burn more calories than you consume, there is no way around this. Your body needs energy constantly. It needs a certain amount of calories or fuel just for your body to function. Your heart needs fuel to beat, your lungs need fuel to breath, your brain needs fuel to function. So just by carrying out these functions alone your metabolism is working and burning calories.

Everything that you do after this basic human function is going to contribute to the rate you burn calories, the rate of your metabolism. General day-to-day activity requires fuel. The rate the calories are consumed is dependent on the demand you put on your body. Ergo, taking the stairs will consume more than taking the lift, parking further away from the shop door and walking further will burn more calories. Even making daily small changes in your movement will contribute to increasing the amount of calories you use.

Bringing regular exercise into your routine will ultimately burn off even more calories. The key is to find the movement that is right for you. Choose an exercise that you can bring into your life and your daily routine with relative ease.

Start by looking back in your journal to task 2 part b, what have you have learned from the choices you made about movement in the past? What worked for you? Why? What didn't work for you? Why?

The movement you choose will be dependent on your level of mobility and fitness at the beginning. Maybe you have limited movement due to the weight you carry or from a physical challenge or injury. If so please consult with a doctor or qualified fitness expert when deciding on what course of action to take.

The key to making any new change in life or starting a new regime is to take it one step at a time. Launching straight away into running 5ks, when you have never run before, or into spending 6 days in the gym right away is not ideal when starting.

Like dieting it won't be sustainable. It might work for some; however if you have tried it before then it didn't work. Don't do it this way again!! Learn from it.

Getting the right movement into your life will not only help you to lose weight and manage your weight for life but it also is worth mentioning the other health benefits of exercise.

- It helps to reduce the risk of premature heart disease and of premature death.
- It reduces the risk of high blood pressure.
- It reduces feeling of anxiety, stress and depression.
- It helps to build and maintain healthy bones, muscles and joints.
- It gives you more energy and stamina.
- It helps you to relax and sleep better.
- It helps to keep cholesterol levels healthy.
- It helps to prevent diabetes.
- It makes you sweat which cleanses and revitalises.
- It has many psychological benefits, such as better concentration, improved memory, greater resilience to depression and stress; and finally – of course
- It helps you to lose weight and keep it off.

There are a lot of good reasons to get active. You don't need me to tell you this; we are surrounded every day by information telling us why we should get active. We all know it is good for us and we all know it is so important in losing weight the healthy way. So why don't we do it? What stops us?

Once again the answer is - our mind! The way we think, our attitudes, our beliefs, these all contribute to the success and failure of everything we do.

You now know you have to *Think Right*. Without addressing what is going on in your mind you are doomed to fail.

So what is going on in your mind in relation to exercise? Do you have an irrational belief around it? Maybe you believe you hate exercise. Maybe you believe because you tried it before and it didn't work it will never work, or maybe you believe you don't have time.

Using what you have learned from task 3 part b, write down again what you have learned from your past experiences with exercise.

What were the things you tried?
What did you like?   Why?
What did you dislike?   Why?

Also look back at how to identify your beliefs. Do you have an irrational belief about exercise? What is it? Is it going to stop you from achieving your goal and enhancing your life? How can you change it to work for you?

The negative self-talk appears for most people around exercise. If you are not a naturally sporting person, getting up and doing exercise of any sort, can be a real chore. More often than not however, this is due to your beliefs and your focus. Focus is a huge help in achieving an active life. All too often we focus on the negatives around exercise. "It makes me sweaty", "I need the time to do it", "I feel out of breath", "I hate gyms", "I don't like exercise classes". "It costs too much money". These all focus on the I CAN'Ts, whereby focusing on I CAN creates a completely different picture.

If you are thinking I CAN then, yes, exercise makes you sweaty but this means you are burning calories. I CAN make the time for it. I can record my programme on the TV so I CAN go for a walk and watch it when I come back.

If I am out of breath I am pushing myself too hard, I CAN slow it down to what I can handle and speed it up from there. I don't like gyms or exercise classes but there are other things that I CAN do and things that don't cost any money.

Once you start getting out there and doing something your focus will change to how good it makes you feel. As I described earlier along with the health benefits of exercise, it actually makes you feel great. You have more energy, you sleep better, you burn more calories so you lose weight faster and you tone up.

Once you get into exercise and moving right in a way that you can enjoy and fit easily into your schedule you will notice the benefits. Once you do there is a real motivation to keep it up. Feeling great and losing weight are what will encourage you to keep at it until it actually becomes a natural automatic part of your lifestyle.

Before I got married I used to get up at 6 am and go to the gym before work. At times it was difficult to maintain especially in the winter in the dark wet mornings, but what kept me going was how great it made me feel. I would get into work wide awake, fresh and energised, ready for the day. That was my focus, on the mornings when the alarm went off and it was dark and wet. I would just think about how I would feel sitting at my desk after my work out. That feeling was so good it always got me out of bed. Comparing this good feeling to how I would feel at my desk if I didn't go was an excellent incentive also.

When I became pregnant this wasn't an option anymore and after having my son it wasn't an option then either. I could have made excuses about how I couldn't go to the gym to exercise but instead I looked for alternatives: as you know, I came up with walking, and fitted it in to suit my son and me.

We both benefited. He got a sleep in the fresh air and I got my exercise. I went every day and it helped me to lose 3 and ½ stone. I didn't need to get up at 6 in the morning or go to a gym. I chose something I liked and that fit into my schedule. This way it was easy to maintain and it became part of my lifestyle.

I still do it today, it helps me to maintain my weight and keep me fit and it also clears my mind for the day ahead.

When you focus on I CAN'T in relation to exercise, straight away you are sabotaging yourself from achieving your goal. *Moving Right* is not only hugely important to help you achieve your desired body shape; it is imperative for your physical and mental wellbeing. These in turn will influence your level of happiness.

You can make all the excuses in the world not to exercise but it is not going to help you to achieve your goal. Keep thinking "I CAN" and complete task six, to formulate your new movement plan.
  The plan is going to help you to achieve your goal and realise your dreams!

TASK SIX: *MY MOVEMENT PLAN*

You are going to make a plan for movement/exercise for the next 2 weeks.

Bearing in mind what you learned from task 2:

- o   What exercise/movement am I going to choose?
- o   How many days per week will I do it?
- o   What days am I going to do it?
- o   What time am I going to do it?
- o   How long am I going to do it for?
- o   What could stop me from carrying out my plan?
- o   How will I overcome this?

Now you have your plan for the next two weeks. At the end of the two weeks sit down and ask yourself:

- ▪   Am I happy with the last two weeks and what I achieved?
- ▪   Am I going to repeat the same schedule for the next two weeks?
- ▪   Am I going to make any changes at this stage to improve my plan or review it again in 2 weeks?

Repeat the process every two weeks and you will come to a time when your new choice of exercise has become a natural part of your weekly routine. And you'll have done it in a way that you decided and with which you are happy.

STRATEGY SIX

Keep your focus on what movement can give you.
Keep in mind the many benefits that it brings.
Don't allow your excuses to block you from carrying out your action plan.

If you find you are struggling with the desire to get up and
move, focus on how good you feel afterwards.
Use this to drive you to action.

Chapter 13:

Step 7: Practice, Practice, Practice

"Knowing is not enough,
we must apply,
Willing is not enough,
we must do"

Johann Wolfgang Von Goethe

Congratulations! You have completed the first 6 steps towards achieving your goal and realising your dreams! The final important step in your journey involves using everything you have learned in those 6 steps and repeating them until they become automatic. It can be strange and difficult when trying something new; making it stick, so to speak. Remember you have been practicing the old habits and ways of thinking for probably many years, they won't disappear overnight. Your mind has been programmed to respond to specific situations in very specific ways. So it is natural for it to react in the old way when faced with a specific situation.

You will know now though from your progress using this book that you are in complete control over what you think, feel and do. I said at the beginning that the outcome of this book was completely down to you. You will therefore decide how it ends.

This book has brought you on a journey of self discovery. It has given you the tools you need to empower yourself to achieve your goals. Every decision you made has been your own, every choice has been yours and every realisation came about from you alone. I asked you questions: you came up with your own answers.

Every step you have taken on this journey has been down to you. What you have put into this is what you will get back; but ten-fold. You have learned how to get to know yourself in a way that has given you the answers you need to tackle your weight once and for all, in a natural way. However, anything that you have learned about yourself and the tools and strategies you have used will all help you in any area of your life not just in relation to your weight.

Your Journey So Far

1. In **step 1**, you identified how being fat makes you feel. My words were Fed Up; you chose your own feelings. You identified them and described them. You connected with them so you could see how bad your weight was making you feel. The importance of this step is in identifying how bad you feel because of your weight. The pain your weight is causing you is what will help to motivate you to change. In life we strive to move away from pain and towards pleasure.

2. In **step 2**, you set your goal, you decided on what pleasure you want to work towards. This is what you want to achieve, what you believe will make you happy. You decided on what your goal is. You made it clear and specific, measurable and set a time for when you want to achieve it by. You broke down your goal into small manageable steps. You decided on what rewards you would give yourself for each step achieved. This is the pleasure you seek - you have identified

how good achieving this goal will make you feel. This is what will also help to motivate you to change.

3. In **step 3**, you have used the past to teach you what will work for you and what won't. You have identified what worked for you before and what did not - and the reasons why. You made a list of the habits and patterns that have been in your life and responsible for your weight gain.

4. In **step 4**, you were introduced to the secret to permanent natural weight loss; the Weight Loss Triad, made up of *Think Right, Eat Right* and *Move Right*. Step 4 focused specifically on *Think Right*. You were introduced to beliefs, both rational and irrational and how they have impacted on your life and your weight to date. You now know how to identify these beliefs as irrational and how to change them so they are instead supporting your new goal, enhancing your life and promoting healthy emotions and behaviours. You know how to deal now with emotions, in a way that does not involve eating to hide or relieve them. You identified your top needs and how you can meet them in a more positive way.

5. In **step 5,** you formulated your own new, healthy, natural eating plan. By using the hunger scale as a tool you decided what you were going to eat and you learned how to manage how much you eat. You have learned how eating consciously and with awareness will enable you to enjoy any situation you are faced with in life. Life is to be enjoyed, not to be filled with guilt for enjoying it. By always making conscious decisions around food and eating there is no need for feelings of regret or guilt afterwards, which only serve to distract you from the new journey you are taking to a happier you.

6. In **step 6** you formulated your own new movement plan. You used what you learned from the past to assist you in your decisions,

encompassing what you would like and what you can fit into your schedule.

The last and final step, Step 7 requires you to practice your new plans. It is time to take action and practice, practice, practice.

Have you learned to do something new in the past? Did you learn how to play the piano? How to dance? How to play a sport? How to drive a car? What did you do to learn this new skill? What did you to do to get better at it? That's right; you practiced, possibly every day until you were able to do it perfectly. You probably practiced it so much that it became automatic; you didn't even have to think about it anymore.

You have practiced your old habits and beliefs for a long time, for so long that they became part of your unconscious and they are automatic. It is vital to remember that these old habits will not disappear overnight, but they will disappear. Your new habits and beliefs with lots of repetition and practice will become your new automatic responses and way of living.

Life is full of reasons to celebrate; life is to be enjoyed and lived. While you are working towards your goal don't forget to enjoy every day. Appreciate the small things as well as the big things. Feel love and give love every day.

Reward yourself for all your achievements along the way. Don't belittle anything you achieve. Make a list of all the things you enjoy and that bring you joy; make these into rewards for your achievements. When you reach each step that you listed on route to your goal, reward yourself. Acknowledge what you have done, what you have achieved.

As well as joy, pain is a part of life too, but now you know how to get through the pain life brings. Feel the emotions; it is a message to your internal world. Listen to what it is saying to you. You will gain strength from feeling it not from avoiding it.

Remember to learn from the past, look forward to the future but live in today.

Now take a little bit of time to complete the last and final task, *My Way Forward*.

TASK SEVEN: *MY WAY FORWARD.*

- What progress have I made from reading this book and doing the tasks?

- What changes will I make help me to *Think Right?*

- What changes will I make to help me to *Eat Right?*

- What changes will I make to help me to *Move right?*

- How will I start/have I started to implement these changes?

- How will these changes improve my everyday life?

On a scale of 1 to 10,

- How motivated do I feel to maintain these changes?

- How happy do I feel now that I have started to do something to change how I feel about my body shape, in a natural and healthy way?

- How motivated do I feel now to achieve my goal?

- How strong is my belief that "I CAN" do this?

STRATEGY SEVEN:

We can condition any new behaviour if we do it with enough intensity and repetition. It will become automatic in time, the same way the old behaviour did. Be clear that the new behaviour is supporting the goals you want in life.

"I CAN"

---

*"We often become what we believe ourselves to be.
If I believe I cannot do something,
it makes me incapable of doing it.*

*When I believe I CAN,
I acquire the ability to do it even
if I didn't have it in the beginning"*

Mahatma Gandhi

I hope that by now your thought of "I CAN do this" is turning into a belief. When you start believing that you can do anything, you CAN do anything. I believe there are 2 types of people in this world, those that have a desire to do things but believe they can't, so they come up with every excuse not to and there are those that always believe they CAN and they go on to achieve anything that they desire.

While I am writing this final chapter, the 44th President of the United States, Barak Obama, visited Ireland as part of a 6 day European Visit. He visited his ancestral home of Moneygall and met some of his family for the first time. As a truly eloquent orator he made a speech to a crowd of thousands people in Dublin, as well as to the millions that were watching around the world. He believes, that no matter what hardships Winter can bring Spring is only around the corner, and no matter what someone tells us can't be done if we believe "Yes, we can" then it can be achieved. Believe in your dreams, your desire and your talent and achieve whatever you want in life no matter what the obstacles are that face you.

Now the ending is all up to you. You have taken the steps and you have learned the tools you need. Now it is time to go and do it - to take action. If you use everything you have learned you will lose weight. I recommend measuring yourself more than relying on the weighing scales but this is up to you. You will see the inches come off and like anything the more you put into this the more you will get back. It is up to you and how badly you want to achieve your goal.

If you find that you are struggling at any stage go back to your journal where you described how you feel being fat and how you will feel if you don't change. Also go back and read how you described the feelings you will have when you achieve your goal and what it will mean to you. These are your motivators. The desire to leave the pain of being fat and the desire to move towards the happiness and joy you will feel when you achieve something that is important to you. You will feel such exhilaration from getting something for you! Something achieved with *your* strength, determination, courage and belief.

Remember, achieving your goals and realising your dreams will bring happiness and joy in itself because you have achieved something that you wanted, something that is important to you, but don't forget about all the joy and happiness and love that surround you every day in your life. It's like climbing that mountain; if you focus on the summit constantly, you will miss out in all the beauty that surrounds you as you take each step on your journey. .

Learn from all you do, be clear about what you want but, live in the day.
You CAN achieve your goals and realise your dreams!
If you believe "I CAN", then you CAN!

Be *Fat and Fed Up, No More!*

---

*"I am the master of my fate
I am the captain of my soul"*

William Ernest Henley

Strategies for Weight Loss & For Life

Staying Motivated:

When you want something new in life it very often requires making a change. This can be difficult at times as you are moving from your comfort zone. If you are making a change because you really want to, because this change is a must and because you desire it badly, then it is important to remind yourself of this while on your journey. If is easy for our levels of motivation to fall when we lose sight of our goal and we forget how badly we want to achieve it. Keep reminding yourself what you want and how badly you want it. You will stay in an unhappy place without that change, remind yourself of this also.

Set your Goal:

Whatever you want to achieve in life, make it specific and clear. Write it down and set yourself a deadline to achieve it.

Then break down this goal into smaller manageable steps. This gives you more clarity and allows you to monitor your progress. Reward yourself when you achieve each step.

You CAN achieve whatever your heart desires if you are clear what that is.

Know your habits:

Identify your behaviours and patterns that have lead you to the place you are in, the place where you are unhappy. When you know what they are, you are not at the mercy of them anymore. They cannot unconsciously destroy what you want in life. You can then change them to work for you and help you to achieve your goal.

Get strength and wisdom from the past:

When you are faced with something that challenges you look to your past for some help. Did you face something similar before? What did you do? Did it work? What could you have done differently? What skills did you use? Do you have those skills now? What does it take to deal with the situation?

Never allow the past be a waste. There is much to be learned from it. Its value is infinite if you learn and use it to enhance your present and future.

Practice your new beliefs:

Your old beliefs have been around for a long time. You have conditioned your mind to respond in a specific way. *This is not going to change overnight.* Keep your new beliefs in your consciousness and practice them at every opportunity, when you stop relying on the old ones the new ones will become automatic in time.

Discard self limiting beliefs:

Anything that happens in your head that is not contributing to your happiness and fulfilment need to be identified and discarded or changed. The ones you need in your life are the thoughts and beliefs that serve to support your goals and enhance your life.

I C A N C o a c h i n g P u b l i s h i n g

Deal with your emotions:

Build an awareness of how things, people, situations and events impact on you in an emotional way. Feel your emotions and don't hide them under a blanket of food - or indeed, anything else.

Identify what happens in your life to trigger your emotions, find out what belief is behind the emotion and check if it is hindering you or useful to you.

Always return to your new positive "Norm":

No matter what happens (e.g., you abandon your new choices temporarily, like eating too much on a weekend away), always go back to your new, healthy, positive "norm" that you have developed, and the rights will soon undo the wrongs. No matter what changes you are making in your life remember that one slip does not put you back to the start, look at what happened, and why, and learn from it. Then go back to the plan you have made to achieve your goal.

Focus on what your positive changes give you:

If you find at times you are struggling with your desire to get moving, or your desire to maintain any change, focus on all the positives that your change is bringing you. Don't allow the self-defeating beliefs in the form of excuses stop you from keeping to your plan. You now know how to challenge your beliefs and change them. Maintain your focus on what you have to gain from the changes you are making.

Keep Practicing:

Any new behaviour will become automatic when you repeat it with conviction and intensity. Be very clear that the behaviour is supporting what you want in life and practice it at every opportunity.

Use these strategies to help you achieve your goals and realise your dreams!

Lightning Source UK Ltd.
Milton Keynes UK
UKOW010755300312

189853UK00001B/17/P